Bo Tice

Patient care and special procedures in radiologic technology

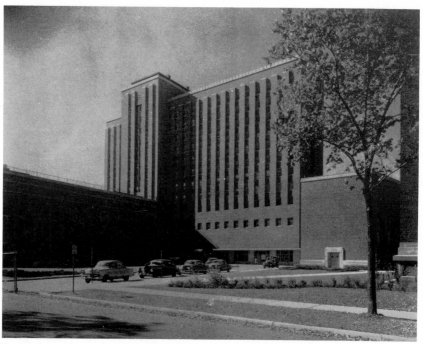

(Courtesy Mayo Memorial Hospital, University of Minnesota Hospitals, Minneapolis, Minn.)

Patient care and special procedures in radiologic technology

John C. Watson, R.T.

*Technical Consultant, Department of Radiology, Yale Medical
Center and Yale-New Haven Hospital, New Haven, Conn.;
formerly Director of Courses in X-ray Technology,
Minneapolis, Minn.*

Third edition

With 148 illustrations

The C. V. Mosby Company

Saint Louis   1969

Foreword

There is a modern concept of nursing which is based on the belief that patient care should be continuous, smoothly integrating the efforts of all concerned, with due regard for the necessary diagnostic and therapeutic techniques. While it is important that examinations be made, it is equally important that they minimize the possibility of inducing or aggravating an illness or counteracting the benefits of previous remedial measures. To reduce the stress on the patient, it is imperative that there be a thorough understanding and integration of all the steps to be taken before, during, and after these activities. This is especially applicable to examinations using radiography. Although many ordinary examinations can be made with little or no disturbance to the patient, there are many specialized techniques incident to the newer procedures (for example, those employing opaques in the vascular system) which require accurate knowledge of the pathological condition being studied, as well as special skills, so that certain results can be obtained without resorting to methods of trial and error and with the minimum of danger and distress to the patient.

The accepted and approved curricula used today in the training of x-ray technicians include many phases of nursing care as related to radiography. Yet there has been an appalling lack of textbook material available for teaching this important subject. The authors of *Patient Care and Special Procedures in X-ray Technology* have rendered a valuable service not only in compiling within these covers an amazingly complete presentation of the principles of nursing care as related to radiography, but also in applying these principles in a specific manner to each of the many techniques which comprise the armamentarium of the well-trained technician. Beyond doubt, this volume is destined to become an integral part of all well-rounded teaching programs, as well as a valuable addition to the thinking technician's reference library.

Alfred B. Greene, R.T., B.S.
Executive director
The American Registry of Radiologic Technologists

Preface

Lack of formal information on the three major phases of x-ray technology has resulted in a gap in the training of many x-ray technologists. This textbook defines the technologist's role in the medical team caring for the sick and injured, supplies specific information on patient care in many diverse situations, and offers practical technical help for doing many special x-ray procedures. The material contained in this book is designed to be of value in the technologist training programs, to supply a reference on special procedures for the trained technologist, and to aid the nursing profession in better understanding the problems of x-ray technology as it relates to the patients in their care.

The continued acceptance of this text is gratifying. In this, the third edition, obsolescence has been combatted by the use of new or modified material where indicated. An additional chapter has been added to the book to permit incorporating helpful material suggested by some of the constructive criticism of the second edition. Descriptions of obsolete techniques have been eliminated with corrected information substituted.

I hope that the third edition will continue to be useful to technologists and students in the field of radiologic technology.

Grateful acknowledgment is made to the following persons for their help in the preparation of this edition: Judith Tyler, R.N., and Betsy Terry, R.N., Yale-New Haven Hospital, for contributions and assistance in those sections of the text concerned with patient care; Richard C. Kebart, R. T., Yale-New Haven Hospital, for assistance in photography and material assembly; Suzanne DeAngelo, Yale-New Haven Hospital, for all secretarial functions connected with this edition; Georg Fridzell, Elema Schonander Company, Solna, Sweden, for use of material in Chapter 8; Hans Jakob, Siemens America, for use of material in connection with zonography.

John C. Watson

Contents

Patient care and special procedures in radiologic technology

Chapter 1

Introduction to patient care

X-RAY TECHNOLOGY AS A PROFESSION
Its beginnings

The radiologic technologist belongs to one of the newer professions closely allied to the medical field. Dedicated to the promotion of health and the prevention and cure of disease, technicians, just like the physician, nurse, social worker, and others of the medical team, have a challenging and satisfying task of serving their fellow men and helping alleviate suffering.

Radiologic technology as a profession had its birth in the early 1900's following the discovery of the invisible, unknown rays. In 1895 Wilhelm Konrad Roentgen discovered

> that a certain combination of a vacuum tube and the application of electricity produced rays which were invisible but which had the power to penetrate solid objects and record the outlines of those objects on a chemically treated screen in the darkness. Immediately, it was apparent that this knowledge could be applied to examination of the soft tissues and bone structure of the human body, and this discovery proved to be of immeasurable value to medical science, particularly when it was found that X-rays affected photographic film in the same way as light.
>
> ...In 1896, one year after he made his discovery, a distinguished meeting of scientists and physicians in Germany who were called together to hear Dr. Roentgen's report, voted that the X-rays be named roentgen's rays in his honor, and the name has persisted. X-ray equipment is therefore commonly called roentgen apparatus, the science is known as roentgenology and X-ray photography is often called roentgenography.*

Subsequent developments in radiology have made the use of x-ray films in diagnosis and therapy a most skilled specialty in medicine. Going hand in hand with the growth of this new science has been the ever-increasing need for skilled technicians to assist physicians in the use of these x-rays both diagnostically and therapeutically. At first, x-ray pictures were taken only by physicists. Then later, physicians and radiologists became the chief operators of x-ray equipment. As hospitals expanded, and with the advancement of medical knowledge, the volume of x-ray examinations requested made it necessary for radiologists to train people who could assist with the technical portion of radiology; so gradually the profession of x-ray technology evolved. As the demand for qualified technicians

---

*Medical Services Series, Bulletin of the Women's Bureau No. 203-8, United States Department of Labor: The outlook for women as medical x-ray technicians, Washington, D. C., 1954, Government Printing Office, pp. 1, 2.

increased, training schools were established where students could receive practical training as well as an adequate scientific background in x-ray technology. Today there are more than 1,000 training schools approved by the American Medical Association.

The x-ray technician at work

An x-ray technician is a technical assistant to a radiologist, the physician who specializes in the use of x-ray and radium in the diagnosis and treatment of diseases. Most technicians work in the field of *diagnostic* x-ray, using x-ray equipment to take pictures of internal parts of the body that the physician wishes to examine. This equipment is also used to detect the presence of foreign matter or an injury and to discover malformation or malfunctioning of various parts of the body.

To prepare for x-ray pictures, technicians position patients between the x-ray tube and the film and cover body areas that are not to be exposed to the rays with a protective lead apron or cloth. When necessary, they set up or adjust devices that prevent the patient from moving. They determine the proper voltage, current, and exposure time, regulate the controls to obtain film of high technical quality, and then process the film for interpretation by the physician.

Diagnostic technicians may also assist physicians in fluoroscopy or other special types of x-ray work. They may prepare a prescribed contrast medium, such as barium salts, which the patient swallows in order to shade various portions of the anatomy to provide proper visibility for x-ray purposes.

Other technicians work in the field of radiation therapy technology, operating special x-ray equipment used for treatment of various types of cancer and tissue infections.

In any event, the x-ray technician's work involves a variety of skills and responsibilities, demanding a background in science, medicine, and nursing.

> . . . . A good foundation in anatomy is necessary in order to obtain exact screening of the bone or body tissue which the physician wishes to examine or treat. Physics and chemistry together provide the technician with knowledge of the properties and action of radioactive substances and of the principles of roentgenography. Knowledge of chemistry is applied to the use of materials which may be necessary to render any part of the anatomy opaque, or sufficiently shaded or dense so that it may be seen when the x-rays penetrate it.
>
> A knowledge of chemical procedure is necessary also in the use of x-ray film and film processing, which the technician must prepare for the radiologist. And physics is important not only in relation to radioactivity, but to electricity, for the x-ray technician is required to know the principles of electricity and the pattern of electrical circuits of the apparatus used.
>
> In addition to using her hands, however, the technician must use her head and also frequently apply some knowledge of mathematics and measuring devices to calculate correct positioning and screening with many kinds of equipment except those which are almost completely automatic. Judgment is necessary, too, in the application of safety rules, although the danger in using x-ray equipment has been reduced to a minimum with the use of modern improvements in protective methods.

From the nursing arts, the x-ray technician will learn about such things as sterile technique, so that she can apply it under certain conditions of work where high standards of cleanliness or antiseptic and aseptic (germ-free) practice are required, for the protection of both patients and medical workers. Proper patient relationships, involving an understanding of, and sympathy for, persons undergoing examination and treatment are also as much a part of the x-ray technician's requirements as of the nurse's.

A certain amount of clerical work is necessary for the x-ray technician's job. This deals mostly with keeping careful and accurate records of all radiology procedures carried out for patients.*

Training for the profession

In most x-ray schools, applicants between 18 and 30 years of age are preferred. Although about 70% of all technicians are women, the proportion of men graduating has increased greatly in the past 10 years. The complexity of the science, the magnitude of the equipment, the technical demands of the profession, and its opportunities and financial rewards are appealing to more and more men.

Preparation for a career in x-ray technology should be under the direct supervision of a certified radiologist. This is best done in one of the over 1,000 schools for x-ray technicians approved by the Council on Medical Education and Hospitals of the American Medical Association and the American College of Radiology. These inspected and approved training programs require that applicants be at least high school graduates and a few require 1 to 2 years of college background. As of July, 1962, any program to be approved had to offer a *minimum* of 2 years training.

Realizing that there is no substitute for thorough and proper training, that a sound foundation is needed on which to build a technical career, and that the public must be protected from inadequately trained technicians, the Council sets certain standards for approval. These standards involve the direction and supervision of a radiologist, a 2-year minimum program including courses in anatomy, chemistry, physics, nursing arts, technique, and many others. They demand certain requirements for safety, an adequate ratio of sick or injured patients per year for a wide range of student experience, optimum facilities, good records, specially trained faculty, and so on.†

The approving boards believe that "the importance of adequate leadership in training cannot be overestimated. Experience has shown that the highest quality of workmanship and the greatest dependability can be obtained from technicians trained under the direction of a qualified radiologist who has been certified by the American Board of Radiology. It is obvious that adequate experience, even under expert guidance, cannot be acquired unless the student too has ample op-

---

*Medical Services Series, Bulletin of the Women's Bureau No. 203-8, United States Department of Labor: The outlook for women as medical x-ray technicians, Washington, D. C., 1954, Government Printing Office, pp. 4, 5.

†Council on Medical Education and Hospitals of the American Medical Association: Approved schools for x-ray technicians, Chicago, 1961, American Medical Association.

portunity to repeat again and again the procedures involved under conditions paralleling those to be encountered in the field of x-ray at large. For this reason it is considered desirable that a training course be conducted in connection with a hospital or medical institution having sufficient volume of work and variety of patient conditions to afford this needed experience. It is unlikely that an institution of less than one hundred twenty-five to one hundred fifty beds would provide these facilities. Even with the above advantages a training period of two years has been found to be the minimum in which proper and adequate instruction can be given."*

Some x-ray schools not associated with a hospital or medical school are commercially operated on a vocational training basis and are *not* approved by these boards. Receiving no training from a qualified radiologist and no practical experience with patients and having inadequate facilities and faculty all mean that the technician graduating from a "short course" such as this will rarely find employment in the modern hospital where scientific advancement demands highly qualified and *registered* technical assistance. They enter the field in competition with highly skilled workers, and their deficiencies are soon apparent.

In the last 10 years there has been a 100% increase of approved schools of x-ray technology, and yet the demand for technicians to fill new positions created by expansion of the profession is such that the American Society of Radiologic Technologists estimates 5,000 technicians are needed each year just to fill expansion and replacement needs alone.†

Opportunities in x-ray technology

While many avenues are open to qualified technicians, the largest number are employed in hospitals, where their work includes all types of radiography, therapy, and administrative detail. They are also in demand for such key positions as chief technician, technical administrator, or director of radiographic technical services.

In industrial plants, graduate technicians provide medical x-ray service to employees. They operate the equipment that is used to detect flaws in castings and forgings, to measure thickness and composition of materials, and to eliminate foreign matter from packaged products. Manufacturers of x-ray equipment and supplies also employ graduates as technical advisors and sales representatives.

Many interesting employment opportunities are available in the United States Public Health Service, the Veterans' Administration, and the Armed Forces. Faculty positions in hospital schools and universities are open to qualified technicians as instructors, assistant directors, and directors of training, and the need is acute.

The demand for qualified x-ray technicians is expected to keep rising, due in part to rapidly expanding hospital and medical programs. The expansion of

---

*American Registry of Radiologic Technologists, Minneapolis, Minn.
†Bulletin of the Women's Bureau, United States Department of Labor: Employment outlook for medical x-ray technicians, Washington, D. C., Government Printing Office.

public health programs and services and growing interest in preventive medicine have increased the number of job opportunities in government employment. In addition, more technicians will be needed to help administer radiotherapy, which has become more widely used with new knowledge of the medical benefits of radioactive material.

During the past 50 years, there has been a vast amount of basic medical research, which is now being applied in the health field. Hospital facilities have been growing, and significant technological advances have occurred in the diagnosis and treatment of diseases and injuries. The expanded use of x-ray equipment has accounted for a part of this advance. Originally confined to bone diagnosis and locating foreign bodies, x-ray is now used in such fields as tuberculosis detection on a large scale, examination of teeth, and treatment of cancer. Routine x-raying of large groups is being performed as part of a program of disease prevention and control by health departments, tuberculosis hospitals, industrial establishments, and health associations in many parts of the United States. All of these developments contribute to a growing need for skilled x-ray technicians.

Financial rewards for the x-ray technician are comparable to those in other fields where longer and more specialized training is required. As the technician becomes more experienced, salaries increase proportionately. A beginning Registered Technician may receive around $5,000 per year, whereas those who advance to teaching and supervisory positions can expect to earn considerably more. Advancement, as in any profession, depends upon the technician's personality, character, ability to assume responsibility, and professional preparation. In general, the technician with some college background advances more rapidly.

Professional organizations

Upon completion of an approved training program, an x-ray technician should apply for formal recognition as a skilled person to the American Registry of Radiologic Technologists. The Registry investigates, examines, and certifies the competency of technicians in the same way that professional medical and nursing agencies examine and register doctors and nurses for approval. Established in 1922 by the American Society of X-ray Technicians and the various American and Canadian radiologic societies, the Registry is the only certifying body for x-ray technicians that is recognized by the American College of Radiology or the American Medical Association. The chief reasons for establishing the Registry were to help raise the ideals and standards of the x-ray technicians, to recognize the value and worth of their training and service, and to prevent fraud and deception of the public. There are in excess of 70,000 persons employed in the United States as x-ray technicians; of these, nearly 60% are registered with the American Registry of Radiologic Technology.

Examinations for registration are held semiannually throughout the United States during the first weekend in May and November. After passing the written examination, which is prepared by the Board of Trustees of The American

Registry of Radiologic Technologists, the technician is awarded a certificate and is entitled to use the title "Radiologic Technologist" and its abbreviation "R.T. (ARRT)," in connection with his name as long as the certificate is in effect.

Any technician who has been certified and is in good standing with the Registry and who is willing to abide by the code of ethics of the Society may apply for membership in The American Society of Radiologic Technologists. The object of the Society is "To promote the science and art of radiography, and to study and discuss all the subjects pertaining thereto." Every x-ray technician should be willing to support the Society in its effort to raise the standards of training and to obtain recognition for efficient, well-qualified technicians. The need for standard qualifications in both personnel and performance is universally recognized. To that end, the ASXT is cooperating with the Registry and other medical organizations to establish more uniform standards of training, standards that will assist in developing well-trained technicians who are so essential to the medical profession.

The American Society of X-ray Technicians was organized in 1920 by Ed C. Jerman. Mr. Jerman, 40 years of age when the x-ray was discovered in 1895, was already an authority in the field of physics and electricity as applied to medicine. He had devised cautery sets and various galvanic and faradic apparatus to be used in medical practice. Margaret Hoing states the following in her history of the Society:

> It has been said that when Mr. Jerman read the first cabled reports of Roentgen's discovery of the X-ray, he was able to assemble the apparatus necessary to repeat the experiment and produce X-ray from equipment already in his possession, with the exception of a "Crookes" vacuum tube. Immediately, he set about to secure one .... As his knowledge of radiological physics increased, he became aware of the fact that physicians who were becoming interested in the use of X-ray in the practice of medicine were extremely eager to acquire fundamental as well as practical knowledge in radiology. The technical service required by both the manufacturer and the physicians created a problem which his training especially fitted him to solve.
>
> In these early days of medical radiology the physician worked with practically no assistants, doing all of his own radiography. As the specialty developed, the routine procedure demanded more time than the radiologist could afford to spend, and it became necessary for him to train an assistant who could assume some of these duties. Mr. Ed C. Jerman, being one of the early authorities on radiographic technique then, was among the first to anticipate the important place the technician would occupy in the field of medicine. With the co-operation and support of several leading radiologists, he did some missionary work among the technicians and found them enthusiastic to form a society wherein they might mingle with their fellow workers, discuss their mutual problems, and exchange helpful suggestions. A pioneer in advocating proper training for technicians, he was the first layman upon whom was conferred the title of Professor of Radiological Technic.*

The Society has grown to over 10,000 members with local organizations in

---

*Hoing, M.: The American Society of X-Ray Technicians—a history of the A.S.X.T., 1920-1950, St. Paul, 1952, Bruce Publishing Co.

each state of the union. Just as in other professional organizations, the benefits are many for those who join their American Society of Radiologic Technologists. One benefit is a subscription to the only national technicians publication, *Radiologic Technology,* formerly called *The X-ray Technician,* an outstanding magazine published every 2 months. In order to keep informed of new advances, techniques, and procedures, every technician should feel obligated to read professional literature. The Society aids in job placement, lobbying, providing studies on radiation protection, and in many other areas. Each year at the annual national meeting, it conducts refresher courses to help technicians keep abreast of the field and attain a higher degree of skill.

The following is the code of ethics established by the Society for the x-ray technician.

The Radiologic Technologist's Creed

We believe that every radiologic technologist should work under the direct supervision of, and be directly responsible to, some member of the Radiological, Medical, Surgical or Dental profession, such member being generally recognized in his profession as being qualified to do the work attempted.

We are opposed to the so-called schools (whether conducted by professional men or laymen) who urge the attendance of any or all laymen with the promise of speedy preparation and handsome remuneration for their services. In other words, we are opposed to the commercial school.

We believe that the standard for all plate and film work should be established by the professional man doing the work of interpretation, and that it is our duty to qualify ourselves to produce the desired standard.

We believe that no expression of our opinion regarding treatment, diagnosis or interpretation concerning any patient with whom we work should ever be given to other than the professional man to whom we are responsible.*

HEALTH
The meaning of health

X-ray technology is primarily concerned with the diagnosis and treatment of illness. In order for the technician to become skilled in the field of helping diagnose and treat illness, it is of first importance to understand wellness, the total *positive* side of health. Health has been defined in a number of ways, but the World Health Organization, sponsored by the various governments of the United Nations, defines it most completely in the following way:

Health is a state of complete physical, mental and social well-being, and not merely the absence of disease or infirmity. The enjoyment of the highest attainable standard of health is one of the fundamental rights of every human being without distinction of race, religion, political belief, economic or social condition. The health of all people is fundamental to the attainment of peace and security and is dependent upon the fullest cooperation of individuals and states.†

---

*Hoing, M.: The American Society of X-Ray Technicians—a history of the A.S.X.T., 1920-1950, St. Paul, 1952, Bruce Publishing Co.

†Hydett V. Z.: World Health Organization—progress and plans, Washington, D. C., 1948, Department of State Bulletins, Publication 3126.

Understanding this concept of health, the technician in her daily work in dealing with the *ill* person will see the importance of her part in helping him to be a *well* person. X-rays then cease to be merely routine procedures. She finds that her thinking involves not only the sick patient of the present but also the healthy person of the future. Because she has a real sense of belonging and fitting into the total health picture, work that could be repetitious, dull, and demanding now has been given meaning and significance.

Advances in health and health problems of today

Although tremendous strides toward good health have been made in recent years, other great problems remain with us. Some are even a direct result of the *solution* of *other* problems. Knowledge and practice of aseptic technique and better infant care have given us a reduction in infant and maternal mortality. As a nation we have greatly improved nutrition. The decrease in communicable diseases and the discovery and use of antibiotics have cut down mortality and have prolonged life. Better methods of diagnosis, including the use of x-ray procedures, increase the chances for early disease detection, thereby increasing the life span. All of this means, however, that *more* people are living *longer*. And living longer means that body tissues just naturally are going to wear out or degenerate. And so it is that at the present, with so many thousands living longer *due* to improved health, they are now falling heir to *degenerative* diseases. Instead of tuberculosis, pneumonia, and diarrhea being the leading causes of death as they were in 1900, *now* degenerative heart and blood vessel diseases are the leading causes of death and claim the lives of thousands. How often we hear the words strokes, coronaries, heart attacks, and cerebral hemorrhage. No one is immune to this gradual wearing out of body tissues.[†]

Living that much longer also makes a person that much more likely to succumb to cancer. More older people seem to be getting cancer *because there are more older people.* This is the second leading cause of death in the United States.[*] Accidents, both at home and on the highway, present another health problem yet unsolved and rate fourth in importance as a cause of death.[†] Even though much progress has been made in the treatment of mental disease and also in its prevention (mental health), yet lack of facilities and too few doctors and trained personnel to care for the mentally ill present us with another major health problem.

Geriatrics, the field of science especially concerned with older people, has blossomed in the last decade. The very fact that people are living to *be* 80 or 90 years of age has demanded that we turn our attention to their physical and emotional welfare. This is reflected in federal and state legislation to aid in the

---

[*]United States Department of Health, Education and Welfare, Public Health Service, National Office of Vital Statistics: Vital statistics of the United States—1959, vol. II, Washington, D. C., 1959, Government Printing Office.

[†]National Safety Council: Accident facts, Chicago, 1962, The Council.

building of nursing homes, chronic care centers, increased social security grants, increased income tax exemptions, and so on. It is almost impossible, however, to fill the gap between geriatric demand and alleviation of the problem. It is one that will be with us for years.

Implications for the x-ray technician

All of the preceding factors, of course, will affect the x-ray technician. Rarely will patients be seen who need care for severe nutritional diseases, nor will hospital wards ever be filled with patients having pneumonia or diphtheria. On the other hand, many more older persons will be seen coming to the clinics, physicians' offices, and hospitals. The technician's work, more often than not, will involve x-rays to help diagnose cancer, conditions of the heart and blood vessels, or arthritis. For with the joys, satisfactions, and assets of longer life also come the degenerative diseases, problems, and complexities of living longer.

Resources for health

In the United States, many agencies and both private and professional organizations are actively working in research and promoting better health. More than 10 years ago, a post in the President's Cabinet was created for health and social welfare. We have the United States Public Health Service, the Federal Security Agency, and the many voluntary organizations. Examples of professional organizations working in the behalf of better health are the American Medical Association, the National League for Nursing, and the American Society of Radiologic Technologists. State and local health departments are also vital for the promotion of health, the maintenance of health standards, and the provision of good patient care.

Not only the United States but also the entire world seems aware of these problems and interested in solving them. The International Red Cross, the World Health Organization, and the Rockefeller Foundation are some of the more important world organizations concerned with health.

But the most important of all is the individual—the physician, the social worker, the technician, the nurse—each with a compassionate concern for his fellow man and each trying in his own field to guide his patient to health.

THE HOSPITAL
Its history

The word "hospital" is derived from the French word *hospes*, meaning guest. Every person concerned with patient care interprets the hospital to patients and has the responsibility of serving as host or hostess. And it is of prime importance to receive and care for the patient as a guest with the graciousness of a considerate host. This is a concept either never grasped or else frequently lost by many nurses, technicians, and doctors within the modern hospital. Efficiency, the latest scientific gadgets and techniques, and time and motion studies seem to have displaced the more important concepts of regard for human dignity and compassion for the suffering of others.

The Greeks and Egyptians founded the earliest hospitals where the sick were gathered together in one place to merely facilitate their care. Later, because of the doctrines of Jesus Christ and the spread of Christianity, there later developed a new spirit of compassion toward the sick, and gradually more hospitals were established throughout eastern Europe and the Roman Empire. The first hospital in western Europe was founded in 380 A.D. by Fabiola, a wealthy Roman matron. During the Middle Ages, hospitals were associated with cloisters and monasteries which not only provided care for the sick but also rest for pilgrims and travelers. Nursing the sick became associated with religious orders, and these orders and their corresponding hospitals gradually extended their work. In the early nineteenth century when Theodore Fleidner and his wife opened a small hospital in Kaiserswerth, Germany, the so-called modern period of nursing began. A few years later, in 1854, Florence Nightingale pointed the way to nursing reform and better hospital management and construction by her clear-sighted criticism during the Crimean War. In fact, she is one of four persons to whom modern hospitals owe their existence. The other three are Morton, for discovering anesthesia, and Pasteur and Lister, for their studies on antisepsis, asepsis, and modern sanitation.

Today there are over 6,700 approved hospitals in the United States. Indeed, hospitals are the fifth largest industry in this country. Some of the earliest hospitals in the United States, Bellevue Hospital (1736), Pennsylvania Hospital (1751), and Massachusetts General Hospital (1831), are still functioning and offering great service.*

Functions of the hospital

The primary function of the early hospitals was the care of the sick. The modern hospital, however, has four responsibilities: (1) the care of the sick, (2) the promotion of health and the prevention of disease, (3) the education of health personnel such as physicians, nurses, medical and x-ray technicians, physical and ocupational therapists, and (4) the development of research in science and medicine. All hospitals perform the functions of caring for the sick and of promoting health, concurrently, as they give service to the public. Approval for meeting good standards of patient care is given by the American Medical Association Committee on Accreditation, working with the American College of Surgeons and the American Hospital Association.

The extent to which hospitals participate in education and research, however, depends upon the type of hospital, whether it is associated with a medical or nursing school, and whether it is approved by the American Medical Association to give experience to medical personnel. Its size, staff, facilities, and finances

---

*Facilities, services, and programs—1961: Hospitals 36(Part II):445-447, 1962.

also help to determine the extent of the hospital's participation in research and education.

Types of hospitals

Hospitals today are classified in two main ways: (1) according to their support or control and (2) according to the type of clinical services offered.

The first classification includes both government or public hospitals and private hospitals. Public hospitals are owned and controlled by the Federal, state, county, or city government: for example, the Army and Navy hospitals, Veterans' Administration hospitals, and those under the jurisdiction of the United States Public Health Service. Other public hospitals supported by the state, county, or city are generally for those patients unable to pay completely for their own care. Private hospitals may be either voluntary or proprietary. Voluntary hospitals operate on a nonprofit basis. Some are owned by churches and religious groups. Proprietary hospitals are owned by corporations or individuals and are usually operated on a commercial or profit basis.

Hospitals in the second group are classified according to the services offered. In this group the general hospital is the most common, admitting and treating patients with all types of clinical diseases. Special hospitals include the nervous and mental institutions, the tuberculosis hospitals, the maternity hospitals, and those specializing in the care of children, communicable diseases, orthopedic conditions, and others.

Cost of medical and hospital care

It is not the purpose of this text to outline the financial problems of hospitals nor the expense involved in hospital care, but as a part of the medical team dedicated to the care and treatment of patients, it is important for the technician to understand the basic problems involved in hospital expense. Although hospital charges are sometimes described as outrageous and exorbitant, they are not too difficult to explain. For each patient under hospital care, many persons are required to render the total hospital services necessary. Nursing care must be provided 24 hours a day. Medical care provided by interns, resident physicians, or house doctors, drugs and medications, food, and laboratory and x-ray procedures are all costly. Great expense is involved in the housekeeping, janitorial, and laundry services, as well as the use of all hospital equipment. Thus it is imperative for the technician to handle equipment with extreme care and by careful technique to avoid unnecessary duplication of examinations. The technician, as well as all personnel concerned with patient care, must consider these basic expense factors and, from a public relations standpoint, interpret the cost of hospital and medical care to the patient. Fortunately, more than two thirds of the population of the United States now carry some form of insurance which makes hospitalization not only feasible but also frequently the most economical way for a family to meet an illness problem.

Organization of the hospital

Good hospital organization is absolutely necessary to provide the patient with the best, most efficient, and yet economical care. Regardless of ownership or control of the hospital, there is usually a governing board, either elected or appointed, which is responsible for the policies, services, and finances of the institution. In a private hospital it may be a board of directors or trustees; in a university hospital it may be the board of regents. Directly responsible to the governing board is the hospital superintendent, who has many departmental assistants to assure the highest degree of patient care. Fig. 1-1 is a diagram showing the organization of a private hospital similar to the chain of command in any other hospital.

THE MEDICAL TEAM
Its personnel

In order to give the patient the kind of care he wants and deserves, it is obvious that not only are good hospital administration and organization needed but also a well-qualified staff who work together as a team. In the broadest sense, the term medical team personnel applies to everyone concerned with the operation of the hospital: the nurses, technicians, physicians, administrators, janitors, maintenance men, and others. However, the two broad classifications are (1) the administrative team and (2) the medical team.

The administrative team is composed of the hospital governing board, the hospital administrator and his various staffs, the maintenance, engineering, and housekeeping staffs. The duties of this group are concerned with finance, purchasing, general business administration, and maintenance and operation of the physical plant and properties of the hospital.

The medical team is composed of the medical, nursing, and technical staffs (physical and occupational therapists, technicians, social workers, and others). Their duties are concerned with the actual diagnosis and treatment of disease.

The medical staff of a hospital consists of physicians who have applied to the board for admission on the staff and have been accepted. They may be general practitioners, who are the so-called family doctors, or they may be specialists. As a general rule, the patient's first contact is with the doctor in general practice. If the doctor believes that his training and experience are adequate to help the patient, he will continue with the diagnosis and treatment. When he believes that the problem requires specialized experience, he will refer his patient to a specialist, a physician whose added 2 or 5 years in specialized training qualify him to practice within a certain sphere or group of medical problems. For example, the orthopedist is a specialist in diseases or injuries of the bones and joints, the internist diagnoses and treats nonsurgical conditions, and the radiologist is concerned with the diagnosis and treatment of disease, using the x-ray and radioactive materials. There are, of course, many other specialists, but these are representative.

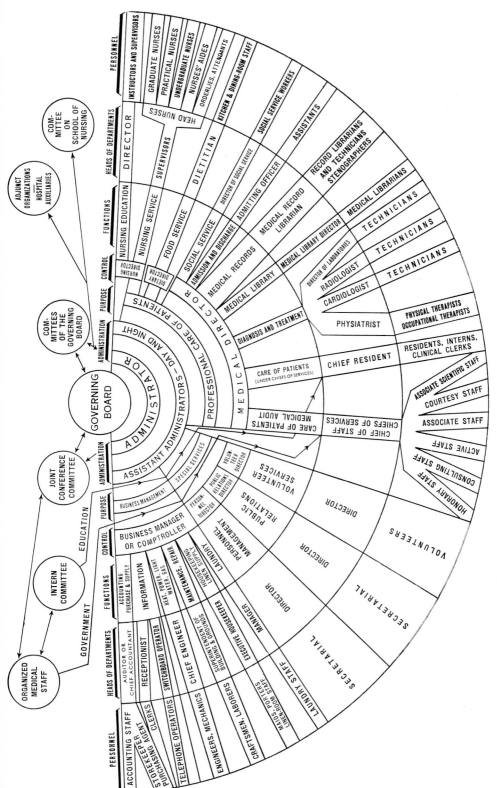

Fig. 1-1. Organization of a hospital. (From MacEachern, M. T.: Hospital organization and management, ed. 3, Chicago, 1957, Physicians' Record Co.)

On a hospital medical staff there may also be resident physicians—those who are specializing in a certain branch of medicine and are actually living in or residing at the hospital while they are doing so. Interns are a part of many hospitals, also, if they have been qualified to engage in teaching programs. Interns are doctors who have completed 4 years of medical school and are in one more stage of medical career development.

The nursing staff is composed of graduate or registered nurses and often student nurses, practical nurses, and nursing aides, all of whom work together with varying degrees of responsibility for patient care.

Responsibilities of the team

In order for the medical team to be effective, there must be a mutual regard for and understanding of the responsibilities of other members. For example, it would be easy for the technician to lose patience with the operating room surgeon who insists upon haste in the development of important surgical films. Yet the surgeon is directly responsible for that patient. He knows that during the time the technician is developing the film not only is the patient paying for the use of the operating room and anesthetic but also there is a certain amount of surgical risk during the delay. On the other hand, the *doctor* should realize that a film quickly and poorly developed, merely because he demands haste, is also extravagant.

As another example, there may be a delay in bringing the patient to the x-ray department, which the technician may ascribe to inefficiency of the nursing staff. However, he must understand that there are justifiable reasons for delay. Perhaps the doctors have been seeing the patient or perhaps a litter or an aide or an orderly to transport the patient has not been available. The nursing staff, too, must be aware of the *length* of procedures done in the x-ray department and not be critical when patients must remain in x-ray for several hours. It is not only the working together and understanding of the medical team that guarantees fine care but also the team spirit—the cooperation between members and their awareness of the role of others on the team.

Some problems common to the nursing and x-ray departments

The hospital with which the author is associated solved several problems involving the nursing and x-ray departments in a unique fashion. A committee composed of three x-ray technicians and three graduate nurses was appointed by the hospital administration to study the major complaints of these departments. The committee mechanics involved discussions of the problems which, in themselves, were very revealing. The committee sought to resolve the problems and carried their suggestions to the x-ray department, the nursing service, the medical staff, and the hospital administrators. The recommendations were studied, approved, and properly effected then, and new policies concerning the two departments made known through head nurse meetings, staff meetings, and other group communications.[46]

Some problems common to both departments in many hospitals are listed below with the views of both the nursing and x-ray staffs and the possible solutions.

Poor preparation of patients. Poor preparation is surely a legitimate complaint of the x-ray department, especially when it concerns examination of the gastrointestinal tract. Often this situation may be due to inconsistency of preparation orders. The "routine" enema and castor oil orders of the patient's physician may differ from the "routine" orders of the radiologist, even though they are in the same hospital; hence some preparations may not be complete enough. Therefore there must be agreement among the medical staff themselves concerning orders for proper and thorough patient preparations and *standardization* of these orders.

Some patients may be *too ill* to be prepared adequately. Therefore, the physician should use the degree of illness of the patient as a gauge in ordering certain types of x-ray procedures.

Another reason for a poor preparation may be the *insufficient training* and *supervision* of the personnel involved. *Anyone*—nurse, aide, or orderly—assigned to the preparation of patients and administration of enemas *must* be thoroughly aware of the correct procedure or supervised until they are, and then their work must be checked by the nurse in charge.

Cancellation of examination following patient preparation. The cancelled examination is a legitimate complaint of the nursing staff, since an ill patient has undergone thorough and exhausting preparation and valuable nursing time has been wasted. Because reports of earlier examinations may not have reached the patient's chart, the doctor may order additional examinations or even a repeat film, which the radiologist or technician will discover need not be done after the patient arrives in the x-ray department. Therefore, prompt reporting and recording of x-rays are essential so that unnecessary preparations and x-ray procedures not be repeated.

Poor sedation of patients. Poor sedation is a real problem for the technician. It may be that the attending physician, unaware of the positions and limitations in movement necessary to take the ordered films, orders an insufficient amount of drug. Also, a particular patient may have a tolerance to some forms of sedation. The x-ray staff may not have waited the prescribed length of time for the drugs to have taken effect. Therefore, the attending physician must be fully aware of the amount of sedation necessary to control the patient for each type of x-ray procedure and aware, furthermore, of any drug tolerance of the patient. The x-ray should be deferred until sedation has taken complete effect. The presence of the nurse in the room to help soothe the patient is often more effective than the presence of someone unfamiliar.

Lengthy stay in the x-ray department. Frequently an ill patient will be taken to the x-ray department early in the morning and may not be returned to the ward for several hours. Many examinations, of course, require that repeated x-ray pictures be taken in stages. However, another reason may be that the radiologists are short staffed; preliminary work can be done by the technicians, but the fluoroscopy and necessary film reading, before a patient can be released, must be done by the already overburdened radiologist.

The nursing staff must be sure to inform the x-ray department of a patient's condition and degree of illness so that, in scheduling, the more severely ill patient can be hurried through his examination as quickly as possible. The nursing staff should be aware, too, of the length of examinations and the problems of the x-ray department in dealing with emergencies, staffing, and so on, just as the x-ray department should be aware of nursing problems.

Attending a sick patient or a child in the x-ray department. The problem of attending a sick patient or a child may be threefold. A station may be too short of nursing staff to permit a nurse to remain in the x-ray department for two or three hours with an adult patient who is *not* critically ill. It is also possible the nurse or aide may hesitate in attending a patient in fluoroscopy, fearing radiation effects. On the other hand, the x-ray staff may be unqualified to care for a very ill patient who has to remain for several hours in the x-ray department.

As a solution, both departments should be aware of and understand the staffing problems of other personnel that particular day or hour of the day. The degree of the patient's illness should be made known by the nursing staff to the x-ray technician. If the patient is acutely ill, a nurse *should* remain with him, attend to his needs, and interpret his illness to the x-ray technician in order to expedite the patient's stay in the department. If the nurse is unable to stay with him, the x-ray department should be informed of specific nursing problems concerning the patient. For example, the diabetic patient receiving insulin, who has had a meal withheld for an x-ray examination, must be observed closely for an insulin reaction. The possible symptoms to be watched for should be reported to the technician. A child, however, is always attended by a nurse or aide from his own station or ward. There should be no exceptions. He should always be given preference by the technician and should not be made to wait unnecessarily. Through various methods of interdepartmental education, the nurses should be informed of radiation effects and hazards as related to them and to the technician, who is repeatedly exposed.

Incomplete x-ray requests. Such requests may well cause difficulty in the x-ray department and on the stations. The mode of transporting the patient should be stated on the request to help the technician in planning the use of the rooms. Most x-ray departments have a room for ambulatory or wheel-chair patients and separate rooms for litter patients. X-ray procedures for litter patients often involve assigning additional technicians to that room as well.

If the x-ray procedure is an emergency, the physician in charge should state the reason on the request in order to properly inform the technician. Great care must be taken to avoid ordering emergency films when there is no good medical reason why the film could not be taken in the ordinary way. When this policy is followed, the x-ray technician, also, must avoid questioning the validity of an emergency request and must carry it out properly and promptly.

Ethics of the medical team

The responsibility of the medical team involves not only cooperation within the team but also loyalty to the whole medical profession, loyalty to the hospital, and loyalty to the patients. It is extremely poor taste and ethically wrong, for example, for a technician to unjustly criticize the nurses, the radiologists, or the hospital. It is even worse to discuss hospital or professional problems in front of patients or in public. This policy, however, does not infer that the hospital and team are without error. If a technician has a legitimate complaint, he or she should work *through* the x-ray department head or chief technician *to* the errant department or persons, quietly, without disrupting the morale of patients and co-workers. When this procedure is followed, it is surprising how often one finds there were other factors involved which make the complaint invalid.

REFERENCES
X-ray technology as a profession

1. American Registry of X-Ray Technicians 1961-62 (circular of information), Alfred B. Greene, Executive Director, Minneapolis, Minn.
2. A basic curriculum in x-ray technology, X-ray Technician 24:218-220, 1952.
3. Careers in x-ray technology (circular of information), Genevieve J. Eilert, Executive Secretary, American Society of X-Ray Technicians, 1962, Fond du Lac, Wis.
4. Conklin, W.: An evaluation of public relations, X-ray Technician 32:500-506, 1961.
5. Council on Medical Education and Hospitals of the American Medical Association: Approved schools for x-ray technicians, Chicago, 1961, American Medical Association.
6. Council on Medical Education and Hospitals of the American Medical Association: Essentials of an accredited school of x-ray technology, Chicago, 1960, American Medical Association.
7. Creed, N. E.: Comparison of curricula in collegiate programs in radiologic technology, X-ray Technician 31:489-497, 1960.
8. Greene, A. B.: The Registry comes of age, X-ray Technician 15:149-153, 192-196, 237-239. 16:25-28, 1944. (Reprinted circular available.)
9. Hoing, M.: The American Society of X-Ray Technicians—a history of the A.S.X.T., 1920-1950, St. Paul, 1952, Bruce Publishing Co.
10. Hoing, M.: The American Society of X-ray Technicians—a history of the A.S.X.T., 1950-1960, vol. II, St. Paul, 1960, Bruce Publishing Co.
11. McClenahan, J.: The role of demons in clinical radiology, X-ray Technician 32:496-499, 1961.
12. Medical Services Series, Bulletin of the Women's Bureau No. 203-8, United States Department of Labor: The outlook for women as medical x-ray technicians, Washington, D. C., 1954, Government Printing Office.
13. Women's Bureau, United States Department of Labor: Employment outlook for medical x-ray technicians, In Women's Bureau, United States Department of Labor: Occupational outlook handbook, Washington, D. C., 1961, Government Printing Office.
14. Olden, R. A.: The technologist of tomorrow, X-ray Technician 24:428, 1953.
15. Smith, C. W.: The x-ray technician of 1900—his problems and apparatus, X-ray Technician 24:278, 1952.
16. Watson, J. C.: Different approach to x-ray training, X-ray Technician 25:42, 1953.

17. Watson, J. C.: Survey of x-ray training programs operated by university medical schools and colleges, X-ray Technician **27**:270, 1956.
18. X-ray—the career for you? (circular of information), Genevieve J. Eilert, Executive Secretary, American Society of X-ray Technicians, Fond du Lac, Wis.

Health

19. Building America's health—findings and recommendations, vol. I, A report to the President by the President's Commission on the Health Needs of the Nation, Washington, D. C., 1953, Government Printing Office.
20. Colcord, J. C.: Your community: its provision for health education, safety and welfare, New York, 1947, Russell Sage Foundation.
21. Dakin, F., and Thompson, E.: Simplified nursing, ed. 7, Philadelphia, 1960, J. B. Lippincott Co., pp. 37-44.
22. Ewing, O. R.: The nation's health: A ten year program, Report to the President, Washington, D. C., 1948, United States Federal Security Agency.
23. Harmer, B., and Henderson, V.: Textbook of the principles and practices of nursing, New York, 1955, The Macmillan Co., pp. 21-55.
24. Hydett, V. Z.: World Health Organization—progress and plans, Washington, D. C., 1948, Department of State Bulletins, Publication 3126.
25. Mather, J. M.: Trends in community health services, Canad. J. Public Health **41**:381, 1950.
26. Montag, M. L., and Swenson, R. P. S.: Fundamentals in nursing care, ed. 3, Philadelphia, 1959, W. B. Saunders Co., chap. 3.
27. Mountain, J. W.: A guide to health organization in the United States, Washington, D. C., 1946, Public Health Service in the Federal Security Agency.
28. United States Department of Health, Education and Welfare, Public Health Service, National Office of Vital Statistics: Vital statistics of the United States—1959, vol. II, Government Printing Office.
29. Reed, L. J.: Local responsibility for world health, Amer. J. Public Health **48**:1363-1367, 1950.
30. Sanai, N.: Health insurance in the United States, New York, 1946, The Commonwealth Fund.

The hospital

31. Bachmeyer, A. C., and Hartman, G., editors: The hospital in modern society, New York, 1943, The Commonwealth Fund.
32. Commission on Hospital Care: Hospital care in the United States, New York, 1947, The Commonwealth Fund.
33. George, F. L., and Kuehn, R. P.: Patterns of patient care, New York, 1955, The Macmillan Co.
34. Harmer, B., and Henderson, V.: Textbook of the principles and practices of nursing, New York, 1955, The Macmillan Co., pp. 56-73.
35. Hawley, P. R.: The responsibility for medical care, Hosp. Prog. **29**:282-284, 1948.
36. Facilities, services, and programs—1961, Hospitals **36**(Part II):444-447, 1962.
37. MacEachern, M. T.: Hospital organization and management, ed. 3, Chicago, Physicians Record Co., pp. 1-27, 29-39, 41-82, 83-124.
38. Montag, M. L., and Swenson, R. P. S.: Fundamentals in nursing care, ed. 3, Philadelphia, 1959, W. B. Saunders Co., chap. 27.
39. Orbison, K.: A handbook of nurse's aides, New York, 1943, Devin-Adair Co., pp. 6-19, 165-168, 189-195.
40. Wright, M. J.: The improvement of patient care, New York, 1954, G. P. Putnam's Sons.

The medical team

41. Boyle, R.: X-ray students learn nursing procedures, X-ray Technician **27**:326, 1956.
42. Craig, A.: Are you an ambassador of good will? Canad. Hosp. **27**:31, 1950.

43. Cunningham, M. L.: Nursing aspects of radiologic technology, X-ray Technician **22:**15, 1950.
44. Densford, K. J., and Everett, M. S.: Ethics for modern nurses—professional ethics I., Philadelphia, 1947, W. B. Saunders Co.
45. Post, J. W.: Medical legal responsibility of the technician, X-ray Technician **24:**17, 1952.
46. Report of Nursing and X-ray Committee (Glen R. Mitchell, Chairman), Mayo Memorial Hospitals, Minneapolis, Minn., April 27, 1956.
47. Spalding, E. K.: Professional nursing—trends and adjustments, ed. 4, Philadelphia, 1950, J. B. Lippincott Co., pp. 477-486.

Chapter 2

The technician and the patient

THE PATIENT'S ILLNESS AND ITS DETERMINATION

The x-ray technician may well ask, "What are these patients like? What symptoms will they have? I know they are usually ill, and I know my job is to help diagnose their illness, but how do I *know* they are sick? And how can I help them?"

Subjective symptoms

The symptoms that the patient may discuss with the technician as he is being prepared for an x-ray procedure, with the nurse during care, or with the physician as he is taking the patient's history are called subjective symptoms. They are symptoms the patient himself feels and knows. Some examples are dizziness, often called vertigo, anorexia, or loss of appetite, perhaps with a resulting weight loss and weakness, nausea or vomiting, and an unsteady gait. The patient may complain of diarrhea, constipation, or any other change in his bowel habits. He may have had a cough for a long time, or he may have coughed or vomited blood. He may have voided blood or noticed some in the stools. Most frequently, however, it is pain as a subjective symptom that brings a patient to a physician to be diagnosed. Strangely enough, even though pain is a danger signal and a sign of something wrong, many persons fear what the physician will tell them, dread surgery and treatment, and therefore delay going to their physician, which can be disastrous. As a member of the medical team, it is the responsibility of the technician, just as it is of the nurse and physician, to encourage persons to seek medical help if any pain persists or if any unusual symptom appears. These then are subjective symptoms, ones that the patient experiences himself.

Objective signs

Physical diagnosis. The objective signs, discovered by the physician as a result of his examination, are called physical signs. Those discovered by the various laboratories and the x-ray department are called laboratory signs.

The physician uses four methods in his physical examination. One is visual *inspection*, or looking. By doing this, he can determine the color, size, shape, position, and movements of many parts of the body and can observe whether they are normal. With special instruments he can inspect the interior of such organs as the eye, trachea, bronchi, stomach, bladder, and rectum. He may see, for example, that a patient's color is not normal, that he is blue or cyanotic; or with the aid of an ophthalmoscope he may see that certain vessels are enlarged on the retina of the eye.

The second method is *palpation,* or feeling. By palpation the physician can determine the size, shape, and position of various internal organs such as the liver, spleen, uterus, or prostate.

The third method used by physicians to determine illness is *percussion,* or striking, a procedure which consists of tapping certain portions of the body and then listening to the sound produced or watching the resultant movement. It is valuable in examination of the lungs, since the ribs and bony covering make the chest inaccessible to palpation and inspection. It is used to determine the presence of certain reflexes, the one at the knee being familiar to everyone.

The fourth method used in physical diagnosis is *auscultation,* or listening, which consists of placing the stethoscope against the body and studying the sounds that are produced.

A great number of objective signs may be discovered through the physical examination, using these four methods, and by general observation of the patient. Some indications of illness may be a fever, a rapid or slow pulse, or a high or low blood pressure. Memory loss, confusion as to time or place (called disorientation), depression or, conversely, hyperactivity, and many more signs can be discovered by physical examination, general observation, or by study of the patient's history.

Laboratory diagnosis. The symptoms discovered by the laboratories and x-ray department, called laboratory signs, are valuable also in telling the medical team what is wrong with the patient. Testing the patient's urine will show whether the urine is acid or alkaline; will indicate its weight as compared to water; or will detect the presence of sugar, bile, or red or white blood cells. In examination of the stool the color, consistency, or presence of blood, pus, or parasites are determined.

The routine blood count examination tells the physician the number of red and white cells in the patient's blood, the kinds of white cells, and the amount of hemoglobin. Evidence of over-radiation would show a decrease in white blood cells. This is a routine examination of patients receiving radiation therapy.

The x-ray department and the technician are as vitally concerned as are the laboratories and the physician in discovering objective signs. The manner in which the technician helps is described later with each special x-ray procedure. These, then, are the ways the medical team knows that the patient is ill; these, then, are the patient's symptoms and signs of illness and the ways by which they may be determined.

"WHAT IS MY PATIENT LIKE?"
The hospital as a determining factor

A great factor in determining the emotional, physical, and economic condition of a patient is the *type* of hospital to which he comes. For example, the patients are happy and generally cheerful in an *obstetric* hospital, since illness is at a minimum and birth is a normal, joyous process. The patients in a hospital that is a large research center for cancer could well be worried. The hospital in a *rural* area may have patients with problems different from those of patients in a city hospital. Their worries could concern their farms and the care of their crops in their absence. Patients in an *urban* hospital may be more concerned with the higher cost of hospital care. Patients in a *public* hospital are sometimes in a lower economic and social group than those in a *private* hospital. They may have language difficulties in making themselves understood or may be more concerned over their children's care during their absence, simply because they cannot afford adequate care for them. And a *children's* hospital would have a wholly different set of conditioning factors, for instance, as compared to a *veterans'* hospital.

While it is dangerous to make false assumptions or clear-cut generalizations, it does behoove x-ray technicians to be fully aware of the hospital they are working in and to analyze the factors that will condition patient reactions. As a result, they will be far more able and prepared to meet the individual needs of the patient.

The whole patient

Regardless of the type of hospital to which the patient comes, however, the technician, like others of the medical team, must not think of him as a "case," as the "second GI series this morning," nor should he slip into the habit of saying, "I've got an angiogram waiting," or "401 has a headache." The patient must *always* be regarded as a *person,* as a human being, not as a "case"; as a person with a home, a family, problems, joys, sorrows, habits, and beliefs similar to those of the technician, the physician, or the nurse. He must never be treated haphazardly, flippantly, or impatiently, but instead graciously by all members of the medical team. As was stated previously, they are the hosts and hostesses of a hospital. They are there primarily to serve the patient, *not* to learn x-ray technology or to earn a salary (Fig. 2-1).

Far too often, members of the medical team shed their manners behind the facade of hospital anonymity. The courtesy with which they would *ordinarily* extend to someone any other place and the awareness of the person as a fellow being are dropped in a hospital. The roles of "all business," "get the work done," or "cool efficiency" are assumed, with the busyness of the hospital and its impersonality used as excuses. Unfortunately, no one is happy, least of all the patient, whose identity seems to be swallowed up. But neither are the technician and nurse who are not maximizing all the gifts of their profession and personalities to extend *optimum* whole patient care.

Patient reactions

Regardless of the patient's condition, his symptoms, or his prognosis, it is the rare patient who is not a little upset and afraid of coming to the hospital.

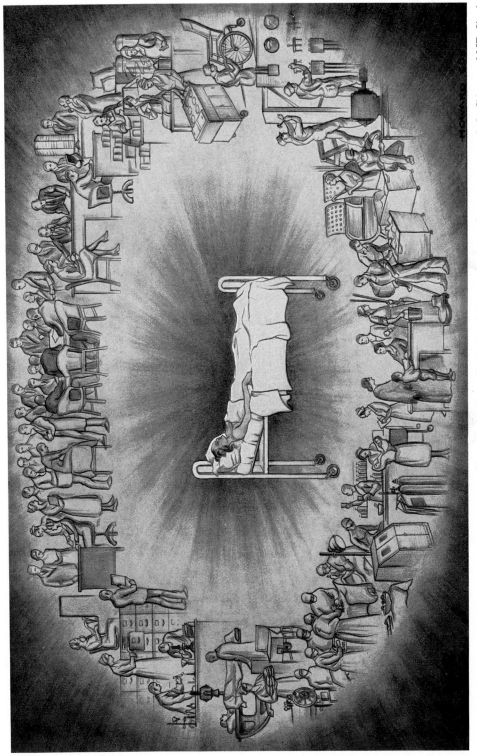

Fig. 2-1. The medical team with the patient as the center. (From MacEachern, M. T.: Hospital organization and management, ed. 3, Chicago, 1957, Physicians' Record Co.)

To the average patient even an x-ray examination is an unusual situation. His apprehension may be due to the fact that he has had no past experience with the type of examination contemplated. It may be the result of other diagnostic procedures where he suffered pain or indignity. Or it could be the result of rumors heard from other patients who have had similar examinations. In any event, the technician can imagine what the patient feels like by asking, "How did I feel on my first day in an x-ray department, or the first day I began my study of x-ray technology, or the first time I was taken on a tour of a hospital, or the first time I helped with a spinogram?" An overall sensation of excitment, fear, and worry may be remembered. The technician may have been pale and trembling or may have had cold, clammy hands or an upset stomach. After he has become familiar with the noise and confusion of a hospital, doctor's office, or clinic, after seeing many people coming and going, and after the sounds and sight of an x-ray machine are no longer frightening, it is hard for him to recall those situations as they were experienced the first time. However, it is imperative that everyone in the medical field remember his own reactions to noise, looming equipment, sickness, and confusion, in order that he may more fully understand his patient's reactions to them. It must be remembered that if these situations frighten well or even medically trained people, they will surely have an impact on those who are sick and uninitiated to hospital atmosphere.

Sometimes, instead of fear reactions, patients will display anger, vented not only because a disease, they feel, has been injustly inflicted upon them but also because they are masking less stoical traits. Hiding behind the mask of rudeness or disgruntlement, the patient feels more "safe" and accepted than if he gave way to his true feelings of despair.

Whatever the patient's reaction is—fear, anger, depression, worry, or despair—all of us in the medical field must try to be understanding, not label a reaction as right or wrong, out of place, or out of proportion, but rather accept it as part of the response of the "whole" patient.

The patient as a controlling factor in x-ray procedures

The ultimate goal of the x-ray technician is the reproduction of a radiograph encompassing in proper balance the factors of good density, a minimum of distortion, proper contrast, and optimum detail, all to be attained with the least distress to the patient. However, in effecting this goal, the patient is often the controlling factor. Since this is so, it is one more reason why the technician must have an understanding of him and how he feels or reacts. An increase in the rate of breathing, trembling, or other symptoms could affect a film, resulting in lack of detail. This, in turn, could lead the radiologist to incorrect findings when reading the film. It is therefore apparent that gaining the confidence of the patient, allaying his fears, and anticipating and responding to his reactions are definitely a part of good x-ray technique.

When a person understands what is expected of him, what to expect from the procedure, and what the consequence of error is, he is less apprehensive and much more cooperative. He is a definite factor in the technical quality of a film. The primary step for the x-ray technician is to establish a good personal relationship with the patient, regard him as a person, take the time to explain the procedure to him, and make him feel that his examination is a joint effort. The success of the examination depends not only upon the technician but also upon the patient.

PATIENT-TECHNICIAN RELATIONSHIPS
Establishing rapport and gaining the patient's confidence

The attitude and manner of the technician. It is often the little things done for the patient that are best remembered and appreciated. Calling a patient by his name, being kind and friendly, giving him a warm smile, and introducing oneself to him can do much to put him at ease and make him feel comfortable and wanted. On the other hand, impatience when talking to a person hard of hearing, loud talking, or evidence of superiority or boredom can fill a patient with doubts about the type of hospital or office to which he has come. A hurried, brusque manner or a bored attitude must be avoided always, although it is often difficult when doctors may be rushing the technician for films, or the schedule is delayed because of unforseen emergencies.

The technician must also avoid any nonpertinent conversation with another technician in front of the patient. The conversation might well involve something entirely foreign to the situation, leaving the patient with a lonely, lost feeling. The only sure way to feel at ease is to be included in what is happening. In any x-ray procedure, the patient *must* be the center of interest and must be a part of what is going on around him. He must be included in all the conversation, even though it is casual, in order to help him be comfortable and cooperative. His whole conception of the hospital or the doctor may be colored by the technicians' graciousness or lack of it.

Much can be said for a warm friendly feeling between a member of the medical team and the patient. Rapport is defined as a relationship of sympathy and confidence. When a technician is in rapport with a patient, both individuals are well satisfied, and a happier situation results. Too often a medical team member is too bound up in his own immediate problems, too involved with himself, and too tied up with the moment to break apart from his own myopic viewpoints and, as a result, fails to reach out and establish a mutual ground for sympathy with his patient. "Feeling into" a situation, called empathy, means putting one's self in the patient's place, being understanding and kind despite irritating distractions of the moment and interest in one's self.

Being a good listener is a quality all medical personnel could develop. We often shut off the gate to conversation by reassuring the patient. When actually *he* may desperately want to unburden himself of his problem or concerns, we cut him off, allay his fears, or reassure him by cheering him up, changing the subject, or handing him a magazine to read. Assuming cheerful, cool nonchalance and saying, "Don't worry," to a patient immersed in worries is shallow and thoughtless. What he needs at that point is a friend—you, the technician, who will look at him, accept him for what he is, and *listen*.

There will be times when the technician will see very disturbing things; for example, a patient with an amputation, a colostomy, an unclean body, or a victim of a severe accident. Frequently the patient is aware of the reaction he causes and is hypersensitive to others' feelings about himself. The courteous thing for the technician to do is not to show distaste or displeasure, but, rather, discount the distasteful exterior of the patient and try to see and concentrate on the inner person, a real effort at times.

Not only will there be distasteful situations but also humorous ones. The construction of the human body does not lend itself readily to posing for many types of radiographs. Very often it requires ludicrous positions of the body in order to record some section of the body properly. Persons will react in various ways to this requirement of proper technique. Some patients, with the ability to be amused at their own discomforts, may well, by word or deed, transmit this amusement to the technician. However, the technician must never laugh at a patient or with a patient about anything which is routine in an examination. No one truly enjoys being the center of what he considers a ridiculous situation.

The opposite of the patient who sees humor in his predicament is the one who becomes indignant at what he may well consider to be a senseless imposition. Firmness can be tempered with an explanation and a reason, but again the patient is a contributing factor to the quality of the film. Learning to control personal emotions, thereby contributing to the patient's ability to control his reactions, is a great step toward becoming a good technician.

Explanation of a procedure. Explanation of a procedure to a patient can be easily overlooked in the technician's haste and preoccupation, especially if it is one which is commonly done. Although the technician has taken hundreds of one particular x-ray picture, it may well be the first time the patient has had one, or even the first time he has been in a hospital. Nothing must be taken for granted, and the most simple procedures must be explained. The technician should gauge the explanation according to the age of the patient, the degree of his illness, his intelligence, and any language difficulties. For instance, it would be pointless to undertake an involved explanation to a semiconscious or a senile patient or a 6-year-old child. It is generally a good idea, after a technician has introduced himself, to ask if the patient has ever had this particular study before. If the answer is "Yes," the technician may then reply in the following manner: "Then you probably know that the doctor will inject a dye into your arm and that we will be taking several x-rays." If his answer is "No," a more thorough explanation should be undertaken. "Mrs. Adams, the doctor wants to take a picture of your stomach. When you swallow this glass of white, chalky liquid, it will fill your stomach and show up on the x-ray image. The doctor will tell you when to drink it. You will be standing in front of the x-ray machine, the lights will be out, and the noises you will hear are those of the x-ray machine taking the picture." More specific examples of explanations will be given in a later section, but at this point it is important to remember that explanations to a patient not only contribute to his comfort and ease but also actually help the technician. The patient will be far more helpful in following instructions and will cooperate more fully with the technician and radiologist if he understands what is going on and what will be happening to him.

Providing privacy. Providing privacy is another way in which the technician can make the patient's contact with the x-ray department and hospital a more pleasant one. It is fairly easy to become negligent and forgetful, since the technician has become accustomed to seeing limbs and parts of the body exposed. Yet it will be extremely helpful if he can constantly remind himself, "How would *I* want to be treated were I having this done?" The technician should keep the patient covered until the area for x-ray needs to be exposed and then reveal only as much as necessary. This procedure pertains to all types of x-ray examinations, because everyone is sensitive and reluctant to expose himself, regardless of the particular part of the anatomy or the amount of the exposure. It is also embarrassing for a patient to have technicians constantly entering and leaving the x-ray room, because it means that he is exposed to them and to patients waiting outside as the door opens and closes. It is courteous to knock, enter quickly, and then identify oneself to the patient. If a radiologist enters the room, the technician must introduce him immediately to the patient, thereby identifying him as part of the procedure.

Providing comfort. Comfort is another courtesy the technician, as a hospital host or hostess, should extend to the patient. Many patients must wait long hours for the completion of x-ray examinations. Some have traveled long distances. Many have had nothing to eat for hours, plus extensive preparatory enemas. leaving them weak and tired. Although these situations cannot be avoided, the technician has the power to make this waiting period as short, pleasant, and comfortable as possible. He can see that reading material is provided; that the patient is kept comfortably warm and is not exposed to drafts; that he has a place to lie down if he is ill and that he is reassured during a long wait when delay is unavoidable. It is important to minimize long waits by not calling a patient too soon from the station or ward before the x-ray schedule is open to receive him.

During certain x-ray procedures, when it is necessary for the patient to lie on the hard x-ray table, a soft mattress, pad, or cotton blanket can be placed under him. Propping the patient with pillows and padding his bony prominences, such as the sacrum, hips, and shoulder blades, can be effected with pillows, cotton blankets, soft pads, or foam rubber. If he must wait for the radiologist, then it is the technician's responsibility to see that he is sufficiently warm and covered while on the table.

Handling the patient gently is also essential to his comfort. He is often ill and

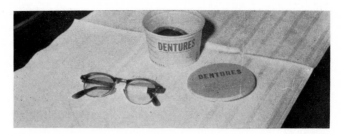

Fig. 2-2. Care of personal property. If glasses or dentures must be removed and cannot be given to the patient or left at the bedside for safekeeping, they should be properly labeled with the patient's name and hospital number.

weak and unable to move as quickly as a well person. It is sometimes easier and less painful for the patient to move a part of his body into position himself, with the proper *verbal* guidance of the technician, even though this procedure may require more time. However, if it is necessary to assist him, the technician's handling should be gentle but firm enough to give the patient confidence. All too frequently, whether due to work pressures or thoughtlessness, the technician shoves or probes or positions a limb or body part with apparent haste. And what appears to be cool efficiency and job know-how actually results in pain or discomfort to the patient or distrust of the procedure by the patient.

Care of the patient's personal belongings. Providing safety for the patient's personal belongings is essential to his welfare also. Most x-ray departments have adequate dressing rooms in which to place patients' clothing. However, whenever possible, outpatients should be encouraged to keep purses, billfolds, and jewelry with them. Occasionally a patient will come in with some special device such as crutches, an artificial limb, or an ileostomy bag. These must be specially cared for in a safe place and not left where they could be stumbled over or damaged. If a patient needs to have his eyeglasses removed for a certain procedure, he should be encouraged either to place them in his purse or pocket, to leave them with a companion, or to hand them to the technician to be labeled with his name and hospital number, on adhesive, and to be put away carefully until the procedure is completed. If dentures must be removed for any procedure involving the gastrointestinal tract or skull, the patient may remove them himself, or if he is too ill, the technician should remove them and be responsible for their safekeeping. The best way is to take a gauze fluff, grasp the dentures with it and remove them, wrapping the dentures in the fluff and placing them in a labeled container until the procedure is completed (Fig. 2-2).

Providing a clean environment

The practice of medical asepsis. A major responsibility of the technician is to protect the patient from further illness. All methods used to control the spread of harmful bacteria and promote their destruction are called medical asepsis.

The medical team must be aware of these methods, since the team is dealing, primarily, not with well persons, but with the ill—people whose natural resistance or immunity to certain diseases is lowered. The technician can surely recall a personal illness that he or she has had, resulting in a weakened condition. A secondary infection, such as a cold or flu, finds fertile ground for growth then. It is in this weakened condition that many patients come to a hospital and frequently are very susceptible to further disease.

The personal hygiene of the technician. One of the most important factors in medical asepsis is the practice of personal hygiene, which can be effected in several ways, some of which are listed as follows:

1. *Handwashing.* Not just a rinsing of the hands but a thorough washing with soap and water should be done after the care of each patient and whenever the technician has had contact with excreta. Handwashing should become a habit the minute patient care is finished, whether the x-ray examination has involved pelvimetry, a barium enema, a pneumoencephalogram, or a film of a patient with an arthritic wrist.

2. *Keeping nails short and clean.* Long nails not only offer an ideal place for bacteria to collect but may also scratch and injure the patient when the technician is positioning him. A nail file should be at every sink in an x-ray department and should be used frequently to clean the nails.

3. *Wearing clean shoes and uniforms.* Dingy, soiled, or stained uniforms and shoes are not only unsightly but are also carriers of disease. The technician must always strive to appear clean and tidy. A patient will feel better and have more confidence in those caring for him if the medical team members present a fresh, clean, and well-groomed appearance.

4. *Bathing daily.* Daily bathing is essential for technicians, with their lifting and moving of patients, busy schedules, and proximity to many people. The use of a good deodorant is advisable. Perfumes should not be used, however. Neither should a technician smoke to the extent that tobacco odor clings to the uniform. Often scents are most repugnant to an ill person.

5. *Hair.* Wearing the hair short or wearing it pinned back if it is long is wise; and, naturally, frequent shampoos not only enhance the technician's appearance but also help to control the spread of bacteria.

6. *Jewelry.* Wearing costume jewelry must be avoided for the same reasons that fingernails must be kept short. First, the patient should be protected from getting scratched, and, second, jewelry offers a perfect harbor for bacteria.

7. *Colds.* Sneezing or coughing into a handkerchief with the head turned to one side or even wearing a mask if the technician has a slight cold not only protects him or her from further infection but also protects other team members and the patient. When one does have a respiratory disease, it is far better to stay home, decreasing chances for complications, than to come to work, exposing oneself, co-workers, and patients to more infection.

General hygiene in the x-ray department. The practice of *personal* hygiene and body cleanliness is a great factor in preventing the spread of disease. However, adhering to *general* hygienic standards is important too in protecting the patient from disease and in practicing medical asepsis.

If a patient must wait in a close stuffy room for his x-ray procedure, his memory of the department will not be too pleasant. A well-ventilated x-ray department, on the other hand, not only makes the technicians and patients more comfortable but also removes the stagnant air and cuts down on air-borne infections. Patients who have colds or coughs or known infections should be kept apart from the others in the waiting rooms for their common good.

Soiled and reused linen is another great factor in spreading disease. It would

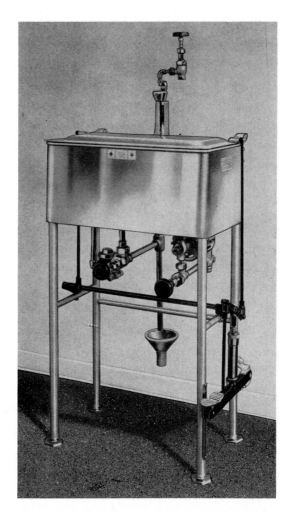

Fig. 2-3. A sterilizer—the type commonly found in x-ray departments. (Courtesy American Sterilizer Co., Erie, Pa.)

be unthinkable for hotels to reuse towels and linen in their rooms. Yet some x-ray departments use repeatedly the same sheet to cover several patients or ask a patient to don a used gown. Every x-ray department should have an ample supply of linen. A gown should be used only once, and each patient should be given a clean one. Sheets should be used only once, and pillowcases changed between usage. If there is a possibility of a pillow becoming soiled with blood, dyes, excreta, or medicine, a plastic cover should be used to protect it before the clean case is put on. Using paper especially made for covering and protecting examining and x-ray tables is very wise.

Disinfection and sterilization. Other means by which the hospital and tech-

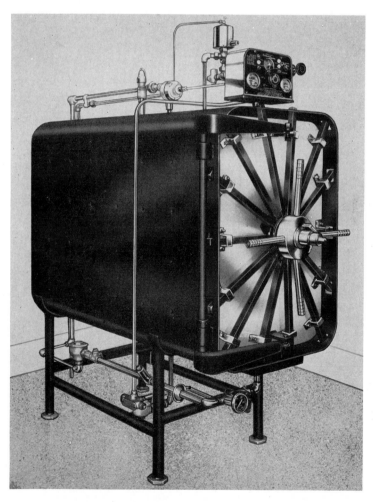

Fig. 2-4. An autoclave, which provides a method of sterilization by steam under pressure. (Courtesy American Sterilizer Co., Erie, Pa.)

nician provide for a clean environment, through medical asepsis, are disinfection and sterilization. Disinfection means the killing of only disease-producing or pathogenic bacteria, not all bacteria. Disinfectants commonly used in hospitals and doctor's offices are 70% alcohol, Zephiran, or mercury bichloride. Good hard scrubbing with soap and water also provides a very adequate disinfectant.

Sterilization means the killing of *all* bacteria, disease producing or otherwise, and is usually effected by boiling or autoclaving for a specified time (Figs. 2-3 and 2-4). Autoclaving involves steam under pressure. The x-ray departments in most hospitals are not equipped to prepare materials for sterilization. Therefore, after using sterile equipment, such as that found on a pneumoencephalogram or spinogram tray, the technician should rinse the articles with cold water and return the tray to the central supply room where trained personnel prepare it for sterilization.

Disinfectants, on the other hand, are used frequently by technicians. They should be used to wipe off x-ray tables after each procedure has been completed. Rubber enema tips, after being thoroughly washed with soap and water, should soak for 5 minutes in one of the disinfectants. This may lead the technician to the questions: "When should something be sterilized and when will a disinfectant be adequate or appropriate?" When should something be autoclaved and not boiled?" The answers depends on two things, the first, whether the x-ray procedure will involve a sterile or nonsterile part of the body. In the barium enema procedure, for instance, the area involved is the gastrointestinal tract and not a sterile area. Therefore, sterile materials need *not* be used but frequently are for aesthetic reasons. In other x-ray procedures, such as the myelogram, pneumoencephalogram, or cystogram, sterile articles *are* absolutely used, since the spinal canal and the bladder *are* sterile areas.

The other determining factor depends on whether the equipment necessary for the x-ray procedure will be damaged by either the disinfectant or the boiling process. Rubber gloves and other rubber articles deteriorate with boiling and are therefore usually autoclaved. Some enema tips are rubber and therefore cannot be boiled. Others are metal and can be boiled. One thing which must be avoided always is the assumption that a disinfectant is all powerful. Relying on a disinfectant instead of the technician's own sense of cleanliness is a common error. For example, any equipment put into a disinfectant must already have been scrubbed with soap and water so that no mucus, excreta, sputum, etc. remain. A disinfectant cannot reach the portion of the tube, enema tip, or thermometer underlying this organic material. Yet, too often, untrained personnel think a quick swish or a short 30 second bath in a disinfectant will clean supplies adequately.

Two words commonly used interchangeably, but incorrectly so, are disinfectant and antiseptic. Antiseptics are not used extensively in hospitals, since they merely stop bacterial *growth* and do not *kill* bacteria.

A more thorough discussion of medical and surgical asepsis will follow in chapters about the isolated patient and the patient in the operating room. At this point the technician should see that, with the practice of personal and general hygiene and through the use of disinfection and sterilization, an environment can be created for the patient where he is not only protected from disease but also more contented and more comfortable.

Providing a safe environment

General rules of safety. Protecting the patient and at the same time protecting the personnel from accidents is another facet of the technician's responsibility to the patient. The accident death total in the United States in 1962 was approximately 96,500, but disabling injuries numbered about ten million! As in earlier years, accidents were the fourth most important cause of death. The accident rate for children is very high, as is the rate for people over 65. In fact, fatal falls make up 55% of all accidental deaths in this age group.* Some general rules of which all members of the medical team should be aware are listed below.

1. By practicing *medical asepsis,* a technician simultaneously provides both a clean *and* safe environment.

2. The technician should learn to watch for any water, other fluids, or objects which may have been spilled or dropped on the floor. They should be wiped up or picked up immediately. It is both embarrassing and unnecessary to have a patient injure himself because he fell on a wet floor or stumbled over something, when all he came to the hospital for was a chest x-ray examination.

3. The technician should remember to walk on the *right* side of the corridors and pass through doors on the *right* side.

4. When transporting patients, the technician should have a firm hold on the litter or wheel chair and should move slowly and with special care around corners and up and down ramps.

5. The preceding two rules apply when pushing the portable x-ray machine also. Looming parts, that are movable, should be centered and not left to jut out from the machine.

6. Cords from portable lights and portable x-ray machines should be gathered up and not left dangling to trip anyone.

7. All hospital personnel should observe the no smoking rules and other fire laws. The technician should know the location of the fire extinguishers in her department and, in case of fire, the exit of choice through which to help the patients.

8. The technician should always be positive that she has the right patient for any x-ray procedure. All hospitals consider it an accident if the wrong patient is given any medication or treatment or radiologic procedure. If the patient is hard of hearing or unable to make himself understood, it is wise to check his

---

*National Safety Council: Accident facts, Chicago, 1962, The Council.

name with his chart or with the nurse, aide, orderly, or relative with the patient, to make sure he *is* the right person.

9. The technician should warn patients of any looming x-ray equipment which they could bump into. It should be pushed out of the way both before and after the x-ray procedure so that it does not interfere with the patient when he rises or positions himself on the table.

10. The technician should be sure there are always enough persons to help with a procedure and should gauge the safety actions according to the age and condition of the patient.

If an accident *does* occur, involving either a patient, a hospital employee, or visitor, a written description and report of the incident must be completed by the appropriate persons. It is then sent to the chief technician, the nursing office, and the hospital superintendent. This procedure accomplishes several things. First, hazards are brought to light and can be removed. Second, carelessness can be exposed, and safety rules thereby given more attention. Third, in the event of a legal problem later, there is a *written* record of the incident and the care given to the person. Such a record is fairer and more accurate than depending on recall or the memory of the people involved. Obviously, completing an accident form *follows*, not *precedes*, the prompt medical care of the injured person.

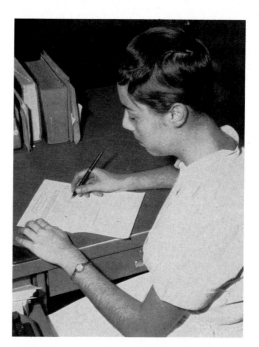

Fig. 2-5. Technician completing an accident or unusual incident report. Such a procedure, by the immediate recording of the incident and the care given, not only calls attention to hazards and carelessness but also is a more accurate legal record than mere memory recall.

A physician must be called immediately to determine the extent of injury, and the chief technician and the station head nurse must be notified (Fig. 2-5).

REFERENCES

The patient's illness and its determination

1. Adams, F. D.: Cabot and Adams physicial diagnosis, ed. 13, Baltimore, 1942, Williams & Wilkins Co., chaps. 1, 2, 3.
2. Harmer, B., and Henderson, V.: Principles and practice of nursing, New York, 1955, The Macmillan Co., pp. 258-269, 269-310, 551-565, 570-608.
3. Major, R. H., and Delph, M. H.: Physical diagnosis, ed. 5, Philadelphia, 1956, W. B. Saunders Co.
4. McClain, M. E., and Gragg, S. H.: Scientific principles in nursing, ed. 5, St. Louis, 1966, The C. V. Mosby Co.
5. Montag, M. L., and Swenson, R. P. S.: Fundamentals in nursing care, ed. 3, Philadelphia, 1959, W. B. Saunders Co., part 3.
6. Hull, E., and Perrodin, C.: Medical nursing, ed. 4, Philadelphia, 1952, F. A. Davis Co., chaps. 2, 3.
7. Pullen, R. L.: Medical diagnosis—applied physical diagnosis, ed. 2, Philadelphia, 1950, W. B. Saunders Co., chaps. 1, 2.

"What is my patient like?"

8. Barraco, N. R.: Considering the sick patient, X-ray Technician **24**:93, 1952.
9. Celestine, Sister: The patient; first, last, and always, Hosp. Prog. **30**:108, 1949.
10. Cooley, C. R.: Social aspects of illness, Philadelphia, 1951, W. B. Saunders Co.
11. Dicks, R. E.: Who is my patient? New York, 1947, The Macmillan Co.
12. Field, M.: Patients are people, New York, 1953, Columbia University Press.
13. Hamilton, P. H.: Patient's families are important, Amer. J. Nurs. **47**:793-795, 1947.
14. Hospital patient as an individual (editorial), Hosp. & Soc. Serv. J. **63**:141-143, 1953.
15. Larsen, V. L.: What hospitalization means to patients, Amer. J. Nurs. **61**:44, 1961.
16. McQuillan, F. L.: The patient's viewpoint, Amer. J. Nurs. **50**:147, 1950.
17. Montag, M. L., and Swenson, R. P. S.: Fundamentals in nursing care, ed. 3, Philadelphia, 1959, W. B. Saunders Co., part 2.
18. Peplau, H.: Loneliness, Amer. J. Nurs. **55**:1476-1478, 1955.
19. Richardson, H. B.: Patients have families, New York, 1945, The Commonwealth Fund.
20. Robinson, G. C.: The patient as a person, New York, 1939, The Commonwealth Fund.

Patient-technician relationships

21. Anderson, C. M.: Emotional hygiene—the art of understanding, ed. 3, Philadelphia, 1943, J. B. Lippincott Co.
22. A textbook of sterilization, Chicago, 1942, Lakeside Press.
23. Bahrenburg, E. C.: Making rubber goods last longer, Amer. J. Nurs. **42**:663-666, 1942.
24. Boniface, Sister M.: Ideal personality for an x-ray technician, X-ray Technician **24**:415, 1953.
25. Brownell, K. O.: A textbook of practical nursing, ed. 4, Philadelphia, 1954, W. B. Saunders Co., pp. 20-31.
26. Dakin, F., and Thompson, E.: Simplified nursing, ed. 7, Philadelphia, 1960, J. B. Lippincott Co., chap. 3.
27. Diehl, H. S., and Boynton, R.: Healthful living for nurses, New York, 1944, McGraw-Hill Book Co.
28. Eliason, E. L., Ferguson, L. K., and Sholtis, L.: Surgical nursing, ed. 10, Philadelphia, 1955, J. B. Lippincott Co., chap. 3.
29. Goulding, F. A., and Torrop, H. M.: The practical nurse and her patient, Philadelphia, 1955, J. B. Lippincott Co., chaps. 1, 7.
30. Gray, A. W.: Protecting patients' property, Mod. Hosp. **78**:58, 1952.
31. Harmer, B., and Henderson, V.: Practice of nursing, New York, 1955, The Macmillan Co., pp. 108-163, 183-229.

32. Hicks, J. W.: The secret of a successful x-ray technician, X-ray Technician **25**:270, 1954.

33. Hylton, O. G.: Safety concerns everyone in the hospital, Mod. Hosp. **75**:84, 1950.

34. Jensen, H. N., and Tillotson, G.: Dependency in nurse-patient relationships, Amer. J. Nurs. **61**:81-84, 1961.

35. Knowles, L. N.: How can we reassure patients?, Amer. J. Nurs. **59**:834-835, 1959.

36. Lockerby, F. K.: Communications for nurses, ed. 2, St. Louis, 1963, The C. V. Mosby Co.

37. Lebin, R., and Manheimer, S.: Courtesy is a special project, Mod. Hosp. **75**:54, 1950.

38. Lehmann, E. E., and Bishop, F. W.: Introducing a better way to process surgical gloves, Mod. Hosp. **71**:78-80, 1948.

39. McClure, C.: Ingredients of gracious nursing, Nursing World **125**:221-224, 1951.

40. McCulloch, E.: Disinfection and sterilization, ed. 2, Philadelphia, 1945, Lea & Febiger.

41. Menninger, W. C.: Understanding yourself, Chicago, 1948, Science Research Associates.

42. Montag, M. L., and Swenson, R. P. S.: Fundamentals in nursing care, ed. 3, Philadelphia, 1959, W. B. Saunders Co., chap. 10.

43. National Safety Council: Accident facts, Chicago, 1962, The Council.

44. Orlando, I. J.: The dynamic nurse—patient relationship, New York, 1961, G. P. Putnam's Sons, Inc.

45. Reinhart, M. J.: Cross-infection—the significance of efficient aseptic technique within the department of radiology, X-ray Technician **32**:487-495, 1961.

46. Smith, M. H. D., and Loosli, C. G.: Hospital cross infections and their control, J. Pediat. **41**:844-852, 1952.

47. Speroff, B. J.: Empathy is important in nursing, Nurs. Outlook **4**:326-328, 1956.

48. Thorman, G.: Toward mental health, Public Affairs Pamphlet No. 120, New York, 1950, Public Affairs Committee.

49. Williams, J. F.: Personal hygiene applied, ed. 8, Philadelphia, 1947, W. B. Saunders Co.

50. Wooders, M. A., and Curtis, D. A.: Emergency care, Philadelphia, 1943, F. A. Davis Co., unit 2.

Chapter 3

The technician and general patient care

PHYSICAL ASSISTANCE IN PATIENT CARE
General rules of body mechanics

Assisting the patient and lifting, moving, and turning him offer some problems. They must always be absolutely safe procedures for *both* the technician and the patient. Such procedures should involve the least amount of body stress for each and yet provide the most comfort for both. Some general principles of body mechanics are listed below to help the technician move more efficiently and effectively without producing stress to the back or body. Backstrain is not due to how *much* work is done but *how* work is done.

> The body may be thought of as a complex mechanism built around a bony skeleton and maintaining the center of gravity and equilibrium by the pull and counter-pull of opposing muscle groups. Any weight or pull which disturbs this center of gravity must be overcome by a counterweight or by a pull of muscle action and there are limits to which the muscle may act without producing strain.*

1. When a patient or object is lifted, held, carried, or moved, stand as close as possible to the person or object. The more the technician leans away from the person, the harder the muscle must work.

2. Keep the arms as close to the vertical axis as possible.

3. Stand with a fairly broad base, the feet about 12 inches apart, one leg ahead of the other, and with the knees bent to aid in balance.

4. Face the direction of weight or pull; the complete motion of moving or lifting should be rhythmical, not jerky.

5. Bend from the hips, not from the shoulders or waist, keeping the back straight.

6. When reaching down to the floor, do not bend, but rather stoop down, again keeping the back straight.

The transfer of a patient from a wheelchair to the x-ray table (Fig. 3-1)

1. Explain to the patient what you want him to do, and allow him to help as much as possible.

2. Always have enough people to help.

3. If possible lock the wheels of the chair, since it could slip out from under the patient as he rises.

---

*Newton, K.: Preventing backstrain in nursing, Am. J. Nursing **43**:921, Oct., 1943.

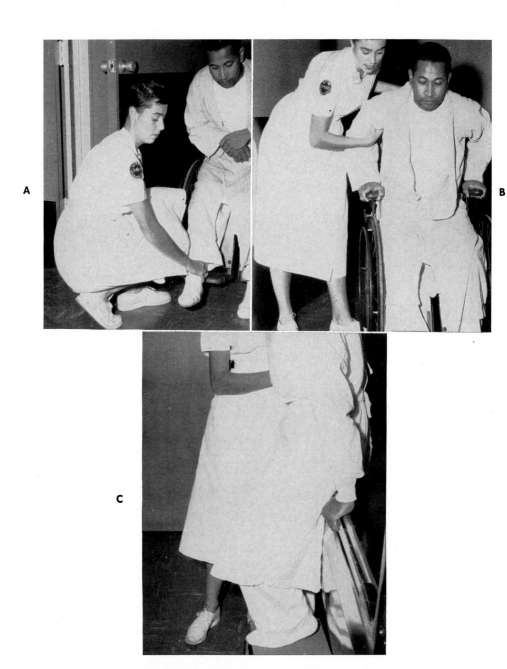

Fig. 3-1. Technician assisting a patient from a wheel chair to the x-ray table. **A,** Stooping down and keeping the back straight rather than bending down from the waist makes use of good body mechanics. The footrest is being raised so that the patient will not step on it and lurch forward. **B,** Locking the wheel chair with one foot behind the wheel, the technician assists the patient up. **C,** The patient is assisted to the stool and steps on it backward rather than stepping up on it and then turning around.

4. Raise the footrest, because if he steps on it, the wheel chair may tip forward and frighten him or cause him to fall forward.

5. Face the patient and have him put his hands on your shoulders. Place your hands at his waist or under his armpits and help him to rise. This method can be used only if the wheel chair has locked wheels. Otherwise, stand at his side with one arm around his back and the hand under his elbow. If the wheels cannot lock, place a foot behind one wheel as the patient rises.

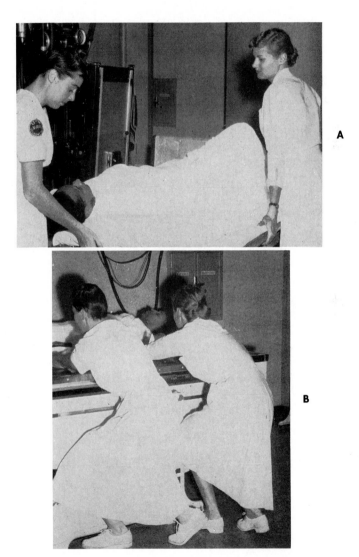

Fig. 3-2. Moving a patient from a litter to the x-ray table. **A,** When a patient can assist himself, he moves his hips first and legs last, with the technicians holding the litter tightly to the x-ray table. The patient is still covered as he moves. **B,** When a patient is unable to move himself, the technicians can bring him over on to the x-ray table from the litter by pulling evenly on the undersheet. Their knees are bent and their backs straight, making use of the larger muscle groups in this procedure.

6. Assist the patient to the footstool at the x-ray table, turn him around, and tell him to step up on the footstool *after* he has turned. He can easily fall from the footstool if he steps on it first and then turns around *on* it.

7. Help the patient to sit on the table.

8. Place one arm behind his back for support and one arm under his knees and swing him to a lying-down position.

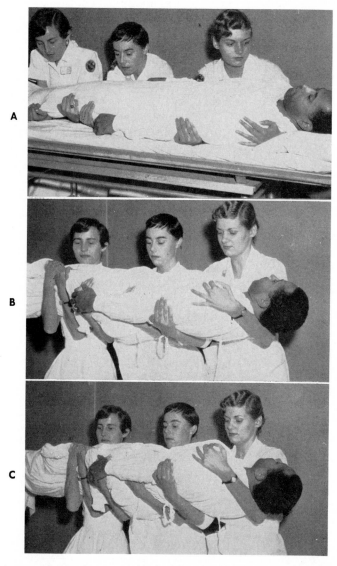

Fig. 3-3. Moving a patient to the x-ray table by lifting him. **A,** When a patient is too heavy to be drawn across the x-ray table, he can be lifted safely. Three or more technicians bend down and place their arms evenly under the patient until they can see their fingers on the opposite side. **B,** On a signal, they lift the patient up and roll him from the forearms back to the upper arms. **C,** The patient is gathered up evenly and carried to the x-ray table.

9. To assist the patient back to the wheel chair follow the same procedure in reverse and observe the same precautions.

The transfer of a patient from a litter to the x-ray table

1. Explain to the patient what is desired and allow him to help as much as he is able.

2. Always have enough people to help.

3. If the patient is able to help at all, the following method can be used: The litter should be placed flush with the x-ray table. It should either be held

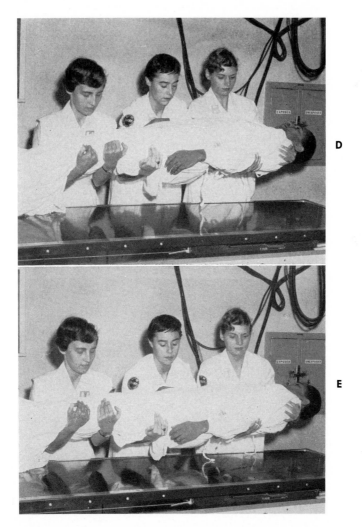

Fig. 3-3, cont'd. D, The technicians approach the x-ray table with bended knees and are careful not to abruptly lower the patient. **E,** The patient is lowered gently to the x-ray table, simultaneously as the technicians further bend their knees and lower themselves.

there by a technician or locked into position so that it does not move away. The patient, still covered with the sheet, can slide onto the x-ray table, moving his hips first, then his shoulders, and last his legs (Fig. 3-2, *A*).

4. If the patient is unable to help at all, one of two methods can be used: First, the two tables can be placed flush and locked or held in position, and he can be moved by two people on the opposite side of the x-ray table, pulling the sheet on which he is lying. The undersheet should extend from the patient's neck to below his knees, otherwise neither his head nor the heavy part of his body will be adequately supported (Fig. 3-2, *B*). Second, the litter can be placed at a ninety degree angle to the foot of the table. Three persons carry the patient over to the x-ray table, one at the shoulders, one at the hips, and one at the legs (Fig. 3-3).

5. In all of the preceding instances, the general principle of body mechanics must be used. If the latter method is used, the three persons must put their arms all the way under the patient so they can see their fingers on the patient's other side. As a signal is given, the patient should be rolled up onto the upper arms and lifted gently over to the x-ray table. In this way the patient's weight is borne by the larger muscle groups, such as the biceps, rather than the forearms.

Moving the patient up

1. Enlist the patient's aid if he can help at all and explain what you are going to do.

2. You should face the patient and the direction of movement, with the hand closest to him at his armpit and the other arm under both of his shoulders.

3. Tell the patient to flex his knees and push up when the signal is given.

4. If the patient cannot assist himself, then technicians should be on either side of him, both facing him, with their arms in the aforementioned positions. On the signal, they should bring the patient with them as they step forward up to the head of the x-ray table (Fig. 3-4).

Turning the patient over

1. With the patient lying flat, move him toward you by placing one arm under his shoulders and one arm under his hips.

2. Then move to the other side of the table and have the patient raise his arm above his head on the side to which you are turning him.

3. Place one hand at his shoulder and one at his hips and gently roll the patient toward you; then flex his knee.

4. The preceding method is suggested since you should always roll the patient *toward* you, not away from you. He must be *moved* to one side of the table first, before he is rolled to the other side, or he may roll off. The tables and litters are exceedingly narrow for the turning of even an average-sized patient, not to mention a large person (Fig. 3-5).

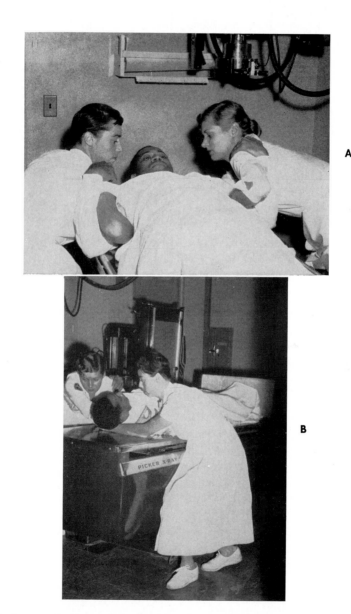

A

B

Fig. 3-4. Moving a patient up on the x-ray table. The technicians face the direction in which they will move. Each places one arm under the patient's one shoulder until the hand is visible at the other shoulder. One hand is placed at the armpit. On a signal, with knees bent and backs straight, they shift their weight on to the forward leg, carrying the patient with them. If the patient is able to assist at all, he can grasp the technicians' shoulders, flex his knees, and push with his feet.

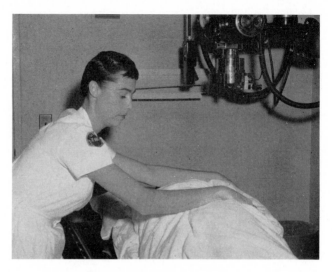

Fig. 3-5. Turning a patient over. The technician always rolls the patient *toward* her, allowing enough room for the patient to turn. The patient is never unduly exposed.

These are some general precautions to follow in providing for the patient's safety and other more specific precautions, such as provision of safety straps on litters, will be mentioned in the chapters about children, elderly, and unconscious patients.

All hospitals have certain procedures to follow and forms to complete if an accident does occur. The value of this was described in the preceding chapter. The important thing is to be aware of the hazards involved in the x-ray department and do all one can to provide for the patient's safety. Then if an accident does occur, prompt reporting to the charge nurse and the chief technician is necessary so that the various hospital procedures can be carried out, certain personnel notified, and the patient receive the prompt medical attention he deserves.

PATIENT CARE AFFECTED BY AGE AND DEGREE OF CONSCIOUSNESS
Care of infants and children

The technician must use patience, skill, ingenuity, and warmth to create as safe and as pleasant an experience as possible for the child. The technician must remember that the child is not only sick but also is in a strange world, away from mother and daddy, his own room, toys, and belongings. He is in a world full of noises, confusion, and haste—with people wearing white masks so he does not even know if they are smiling at him. He is forced into different sleeping and eating routines. The treatment necessary for his improvement may be anything but pleasant. Therefore the technician must surely avoid doing anything further to add to this state of trauma.

A major handicap to be solved between the technician and an infant, i.e., a child below 1 year of age, is the lack of verbal communication possible. The infant probably will react only to how he is being handled or how he feels. This, then, becomes the technician's means of communicating with the infant patient. The patient must not be handled awkwardly. He usually resists restraint. For the first few months of life the child is unable to distinguish persons. Therefore, the properly trained technician may handle the patient with as much or more success than the parent. As the child becomes older, usually between 6 to 9 months, he is better able to distinguish persons and may resist anyone except the parents or others who have been caring for him. As he advances in age, communication becomes easier but is still complicated by his inability to concentrate on any one thing except for a very short time.

Usually children above the age of 5 years make the ideal patients because of their desire to please. The technician who is friendly will have little difficulty with the child who is above this age. Generally speaking, children over 10 will not be alarmed or tense and wary as younger children, because by this time most of them have had some experience with x-ray machines—maybe with routine chest x-ray examinations in school or perhaps for a diagnosis of a broken arm. The important thing to remember is that the hospital can be a frightening place for any child, regardless of age or condition.

Most x-ray departments have a rule to defer calling the ward to summon the child until they are all ready; they then take the child immediately into the room for the procedure without his waiting. This decreases his anxiety and fear. Upon entering the department the child should be greeted warmly with a smile. Perhaps the technician could bend down and take the child's hand. In clinics or offices where the child is an outpatient and must wait for a procedure, washable toys should be provided, such as blocks made of oilcloth, linen books, and wood and plastic toys. In these instances, where the mother is with the child, she could well be asked into the x-ray room too so that the child will not be so frightened. To put the child at ease even more, a technician might show him another child having the same procedure. Praising him for helping the technician or for holding a position usually has good results. Making a game of a procedure is wise too.

The technician should never lie to the child, and tell him, "It won't hurt," when it will. A child must always be told the truth. If the procedure is a simple x-ray of a chest or arm, the technician *can* say it won't hurt. But if he is to have a dye injection or any other more complicated procedure, she must tell him, "It will hurt a little, like a mosquito bite, but it won't be bad, and it won't hurt for long." For the more complicated procedures, the child is given some sedation.

Any child, no matter what the age, sedated or not, should *never* be left alone or with the sides of the crib down. He is brought to the department by a nurse or aide, who helps with the positioning. A child is easily frightened by

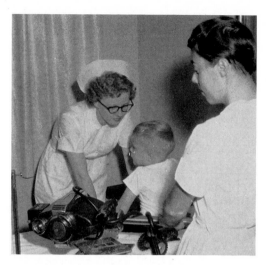

Fig. 3-6. Radiography at the bedside of a child. The technician and pediatric nurse work *together* to explain the procedure and to comfort the child.

the machines and noises and, too, he could easily fall off the table or climb out of the crib.

If the patient is an infant, the nurse bringing him will be wearing a gown and mask and the technician should also put on a mask. If she needs to handle him at all, she should wash her hands even more carefully than usual between patients and don a gown too. It is obvious therefore that a supply of gowns and masks be in every x-ray department. Their use in this instance is not to protect the *technician* from a contagious disease, as will be mentioned later, but to protect the *baby* from further exposure to disease. The baby should be laid on a sheet or nursery tissue, instead of the bare table, to decrease exposure to disease. If diapers need to be removed, the pins must always be closed immediately and put out of the baby's reach. Open safety pins are not infrequently swallowed by babies and such occurrences are rightly called unnecessary accidents.

When a portable x-ray machine is ordered for a child, the preceding suggestions and safety rules should be carried out, even though a nurse helps the technician with positioning and comforting the child. Regardless of the nurse's presence, the technician herself should practice these safety rules and the suggestions for good patient relationships (Figs. 3-6 and 3-7).

Care of the elderly patient

The care of the elderly patient requires a great deal of skill and patience by the medical team. The elderly patient, due to the normal aging process, has some hearing and vision loss, and this, superimposed on illness, can frequently complicate his care. He must be guided and assisted slowly by the technician

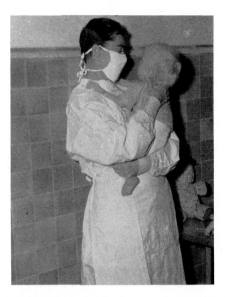

Fig. 3-7. Radiography of the infant. The technician is gowned and masked to keep the ill child from further infection. Her warmth in handling the baby is important in his acceptance of the proceduer.

to compensate for any difficulty in gait and to avoid stumbling. The technician must not rely upon him to tell his name but rather should check with the accompanying chart for his identity before beginning a procedure, because he may not hear correctly if the technician merely said, "You are Mr. Johnson, aren't you?" Because his vision is poor, she must protect him from large x-ray equipment which he may see and also assist him to grasp a glass of barium or grasp the litter side rails. If the procedure involves a recumbent position, the patient must be guided carefully and watched so that in turning he does not fall off the narrow table.

Often poor nutrition accompanies old age. Therefore, when caring for elderly people and especially those who are ill and thin, wise use should be made of pillows and padding to prop the patient and protect the skin over his bony prominences. Even brief contact of his bony parts on the hard unyielding surface of the x-ray table can be extremely uncomfortable and cause his skin to become red and sore.

Patience is required in the preparation of elderly patients since they have less ability to grasp an explanation. They will be much more cooperative if they know what is to be done with them and if the technician has made sure they not only heard but also *understood* her explanation. The technician should keep in mind, however, that the elderly person is reluctant to lose his independence. The very nature of hospital existence and patient care involves dependency. Having everything done for him, everything planned for him, with no responsibility, may not only be objectionable to the older person but also may have an adverse effect on his future care by overemphasizing invalidism and dependency. Therefore, the technician can be watchful of the elderly patient, guiding him and assisting him whenever necessary and in not too obvious a fashion, yet allowing the patient to do what he can for himself, thereby retaining as much healthy independence as is wisely possible.

Care of the senile, semiconscious, and unconscious patient

The senile patient is one who has accompanying mental changes with his increasing age. These patients, and patients with any deviation from normal consciousness, are brought to the x-ray department on litters which often have side rails attached, whereas the elderly patient with no senility may be brought by wheel chair or he may walk. They should be watched very carefully as they are wheeled through the halls. They must *never* be left unattended in the department, because even though there may be side rails on the litter, the senile or semiconscious patient could climb over them and injure himself in a fall while he is waiting for his x-ray examination. The aforementioned precautions about lifting a patient to the x-ray table from a litter must be remembered here as in the care of the elderly patient. The technician should observe the patient closely and see that in his disoriented state he does not fall from the table.

Care of any emotionally disturbed patient

The senile, semiconscious, or *any* emotionally disturbed patient has many apprehensions and will respond unfavorably to any signs of uncertainty on the part of the technician. The technician must attempt to project a feeling of stability and capability to the patient. All preparations for the examination must be carried on as if full cooperation from the patient is the expected and natural thing. Provision for his comfort, safety, and privacy should be no different from that for any other patient. Movement of the patient must be kept at a minimum, however, and verbal directions should not be confusing. Prolonged attempts to gain the patient's confidence and cooperation may well have an adverse effect. The technician should use discretion as to the amount of explanation necessary depending on the patient's degree of consciousness or orientation, that is, the awareness of the time, to the people, and to his surroundings. Again, firmness tempered with sympathy is probably the best approach.

Techniques of radiography common to all of these patients

From the radiographic standpoint, the groups of patients involving variable age or disturbed emotions or consciousness present the same type of problem to the technician. The difficulties that are common to this group are, first, an inability on the part of the patient to understand and follow directions easily and, second, an inability on his part to assume and maintain certain positions commonly required in various examinations. Therefore, the handling of all these patients may require a departure from ordinary technique. In every instance, exposure times must be short with minimizing motion as the object. A departure from the usual positions may be indicated to eliminate unnecessary patient handling. The technician should have all necessary cassettes ready, the technical factors established and set on the x-ray control, and the tube and Bucky diaphragm at the correct point on the table. The lead markers should be affixed to the film, the proper size cone in place, all necessary accessory items conveniently located and the x-ray machine turned on before the patient is brought into the room and placed on the table. The technician's mind is then free to concentrate all attention on the patient.

To emphasize these points and to demonstrate what changes might be necessary, a typical example is cited. The normal procedure for skull examination in a given department might well require the following positions and technical factors:

Position 1. *Posteroanterior*—Technical factors: 40 inch distance 100 Ma., ½ second exposure time, at 78 KVP using the small focal spot of the x-ray tube and the Bucky diaphragm.

Position 2. *Lateral skull stero*—Technical factors: 40 inch distance, 100 Ma., ³⁄₁₀ second at 73 KVP using the small focal spot of the x-ray tube and the Bucky diaphragm.

Position 3. *Occipital skull position*—Technical factors: 40 inch distance, 100 Ma., ½ second at 84 KVP using the small focal spot of the x-ray tube and the Bucky diaphragm.

The use of the described positions and technique would result in films of proper projection and good detail assuming there was no motion or resistance to positioning on the part of the patient. What, however, is being required of the patient? In Position 1, the patient must lie on his stomach with his nose and forehead pressed against the table. In Position 2, the body must be in a semilateral position with the technician forcibly positioning the skull to a true lateral position. In Position 3, the patient is supine, but again the skull is handled forcibly to depress the chin onto the chest. Therefore, in order to obtain proper projection, the patient is required to change position on the table several times, and the technician is firmly handling the skull with each change of position. Obviously the technician will run into strong and continued resistance to this kind of handling from any of the patient types under discussion, with resulting motion and loss of detail on the film regardless of the exposure factors or use of restraint.

What better methods could be used then to obtain this series with little loss in projection or quality? The patient should be on the table in a comfortable, naturally assumed supine position. Position 1 would then be taken anteroposterior, with slight angulation of the x-ray tube if necessary for proper projection. In Position 2 the technician would move the x-ray tube to the side of the table, lower it to the level of the patient's skull, and using a grid cassette as a film holder, direct the x-ray beam across the table thereby obtaining the lateral film without moving the patient. In Position 3 the tube would be moved to a position above the skull, and by proper angulation the occipital position would be obtained without depressing the chin of the patient. The technician then will have obtained all the desired positions without handling the patient except to place him on the table and with comparatively little loss in projection quality.

Assuming that the x-ray machine being used is 300 Ma. equipment with an adequate timer, the technician can change her technique to obtain extremely fast exposure time by the following methods:

1. Shortening the focal film distance to 30 inches.
2. Using an increase in kilovoltage for each position.
3. Using the large focal spot and therefore the 300 Ma. station on the control.

These changes in technical factors would enable the technician to change exposure times from $\frac{1}{2}$ second to as low as $\frac{1}{20}$ second with the result of minimizing motion effect caused by the patient.

All x-ray technique requires compromise. It is a sign of the expert technician when he or she knows when to change from normal procedure to adaptation because of a patient problem. The example described is a method of han-

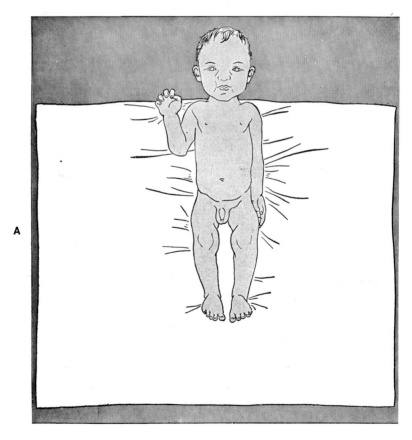

Fig. 3-8. Mummy restraint. **A,** A mummy restraint is a quick and safe method of restraining the young child for treatments and examinations. The restraint should be snug but not tight. Arms and legs should be placed in proper alignment to prevent discomfort or injury.

dling one difficult examination on the patient types described in this chapter.

Restraints of various kinds are sometimes necessary in radiography of the disturbed or infant patient. Invariably the disturbed patient, however, reacts violently to restraint. All other possibilities should be exhausted in obtaining successful examinations before using restraint as a method of ensuring no motion. If restraint must be used for a baby, the mummy type is recommended, but only for the period of taking the film (Fig. 3-8).

In summary, the technician is urged when caring for the infant, the elderly, the emotionally disturbed, or the senile patient to observe the following principles:

1. Have all preparations for the examination completed before admitting the patient to the room.

2. Be sympathetic and patient.

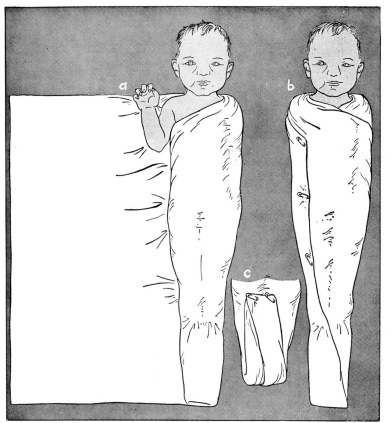

Fig. 3-8, cont'd. B, (a) Bring one end of the sheet snugly over one arm and leg and tuck it well under the body on the opposite side; **(b)** restrain the other arm and leg in the same manner; **(c)** pin the restraint so it will remain snug. (From Benz, G. S.: Pediatric nursing, ed. 5, St. Louis, 1964, The C. V. Mosby Co.)

3. Provide for the patient's comfort, privacy, and safety as you would for any other patient.

4. Work carefully, using ingenuity.

5. Compromise positioning to eliminate handling the patient during the examination.

6. Compromise technical factors to obtain the fastest possible exposure time.

FIRST AID CARE OF THE PATIENT IN EMERGENCIES

At some time during the x-ray technician's experience one or more of the following emergencies will arise. How well the technician handles the situation will depend on his understanding of it and his knowledge of *what to do* and what *not* to do.

Fainting and unconsciousness

The immediate cause of fainting is an insufficient supply of blood to the brain. Want of food, being in a close or crowded room, fatigue, or a severe emotional shock, such as fear or sudden bad news, may cause the patient to faint. The patient who is anxiously waiting for an x-ray procedure, who has not eaten breakfast, who has traveled a long distance to the hospital that day, or who has had long and exhausting preparation certainly fits into this picture. The person usually complains of being sick and dizzy and looks very pale. The forehead is usually covered with perspiration, and the patient may later say that a black cloud seemed to pass in front of his eyes. If possible, the technician should assist the patient to a lying down position and either lower the head or raise his legs with a pillow. Any tight clothing should be loosened. The technician should never attempt to lead a patient who is already faint *to* a cot or litter, however, if one is not *immediately* available. He should instead have him sit in a chair and bend his head forward between his knees. If he is in a place where he can neither lie nor sit, he should kneel on one knee, as if tying a shoe, thus placing the head lower than the heart. Smelling salts or an ammonia inhalant are often used, but generally the patient recovers in a very short time. The radiologist and the station charge nurse should be notified immediately.

An unconscious patient, however, may not always mean one who has fainted. He could be in diabetic coma or in insulin shock, he may have suffered a stroke, or he may be in a state of shock. If he is in diabetic coma, indicating a need for insulin, his skin is hot, dry, and flushed and his breath will have a sweetish odor. The patient in insulin shock, on the other hand, has a need for carbohydrate intake and his skin is pale and moist. The unconscious patient who has had a stroke or apoplexy may have a hot flushed face, unequal pupils, a strong and slow pulse, and heavy respirations. The person in shock, conversely, is usually pale and moist, with a rapid weak pulse and slow shallow respirations. A physician should be notified immediately so that proper treatment can be given in any case.

Nausea and vomiting

If a patient complains of nausea, the technician should immediately provide him with a curved basin, often called a kidney or emesis basin, and a box of tissues. He should be led to privacy if at all possible. If the patient is lying down on a litter waiting for his x-ray examination or on an x-ray table, his head must be turned to the side so he does not inhale or choke on any of the vomitus. This is called aspiration and can be very dangerous. When the patient is weak or elderly, the technician should hold the patient's head to one side, hold the basin with the other hand and wipe the patient's mouth frequently. It is obvious then that tissues and basins should be kept handy in each x-ray room. Mouthwash should be provided in the department, too, since after vomiting it is comforting for the patient to rinse his mouth. If he is an inpatient, the technician should check with the station charge nurse to find out whether his vomitus should be saved and sent back to the station with him to be measured or inspected by the physician. If so, it can be transferred into a cardboard container labeled, and returned with the patient.

Nosebleeds

Nosebleeds occur frequently from high blood pressure or irritations, although they *can* occur spontaneously. The patient should sit up, either tilt his head forward slightly or backward slightly, and breathe through his mouth. Any tight clothing around his neck should be loosened. Cold wet compresses and pressure should be applied over the nose. If the bleeding persists for more than a few minutes, the radiologist should be notified, and in all cases the station charge nurse should be told.

Fractures

When a patient with a fracture is received as an emergency, he is usually accompanied by a physician from the admissions department, so that the technician rarely needs to assume responsibility for this type of patient care. Whatever limb is injured, the clothes should be removed from the unaffected side first, and then carefully slipped off the affected side. The technician must never remove or adjust the splint on the injured area to take the x-ray picture. It must always be left in position and removed only by the radiologist or attending physician.

Epileptic seizure

An epileptic seizure is an attack of a convulsive nature which results in unconsciousness followed by muscle spasms, either mild (petit mal) or severe (grand mal). The cause of epilepsy is unknown, although the disease shows very definite hereditary tendencies in some patients. The convulsion may be preceded by an aura or warning to the patient and often begins with a weird cry, followed by unconsciousness, muscle spasms or marked rigidity, violent jerking spasms, and finally ends after a minute or so in deep slumber. Prevention of injury to the patient during the seizure is of utmost importance. If at all possible, he should be placed in a lying position with a pillow under his head *before* the convulsion so that he does not fall down *during* the attack. In order that he does not bite his tongue or injure his mouth, a washcloth, towel, several thicknesses of gauze fluffs, or a handkerchief should be placed in his mouth between his teeth. Caution must be taken against the technician's own unprotected fingers becoming injured in the patient's mouth. It is wise to keep in the x-ray department a tongue blade padded with a fluff and wound with adhesive at one end to insert in the patient's mouth for this emergency. A physician must be called at once, of course.

Shock and hemorrhage

The technician will rarely encounter shock and hemorrhage as emergencies and, accordingly, will rarely be called upon *individually* to render first aid to the patient. Yet it behooves the x-ray technician to know something about shock and hemorrhage, if only to help the physician carry on the treatment intelligently and concurrently as an x-ray picture is being taken.

Shock is a condition in which all the body activities are greatly depressed with a consequent pooling of blood in the abdomen—away from the vital centers of heart and brain. It follows injury, profuse bleeding, fear, or other great emotional trauma. Following injury, shock may be immediate or delayed; it may be slight or very serious or even fatal. The patient is pale, weak and listless, has a rapid weak pulse, a great drop in blood pressure, irregular respirations, and lowered body temperature.

If a technician is called upon to take emergency x-ray pictures of a patient in shock, he will find the patient in the condition described, with all treatment aimed at keeping him warm, thus preventing further shock and further loss of body heat. In positioning him or taking the x-ray pictures, any warm blankets and covers should be removed only upon permission of the physician and for only a limited time. The patient's position is even more important. Since there is an insufficient supply of blood to the brain and heart, it follows that the logical treatment would be to keep the patient lying on his back with his lower extremities elevated. The technician must always keep this in mind in further positioning the patient. He must never be allowed to sit up for any radiography.

Hemorrhage is the escape of blood from one or more blood vessels of the body, the arteries, veins, or capillaries. The patient in shock from hemorrhage is weak, faint, and restless. He is pale and his skin clammy and cool; his pulse is rapid and weak. The treatment is pressure preferably applied directly on the wound with a clean compress or else at one of the several pressure points. In arterial hemorrhage, pressure must be exerted upon the artery in the area *between* the heart and the wound. To control venous hemorrhage, restriction of the flow must be done by applying pressure upon the side of the wound *away* from the

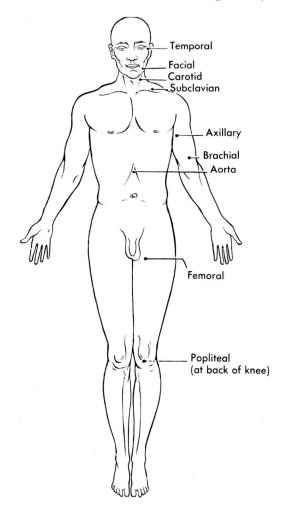

Fig. 3-9. Pressure points. It is wise for the technician and all of the medical team members to have full knowledge of pressure points in the event of a bleeding emergency.

heart. Further treatment is aimed at keeping the patient quiet, flat, and warm. Rarely is the technician called upon to take a film of a patient in this condition until his bleeding is well under control (Fig. 3-9).

Emergency drugs and equipment

Every x-ray department should have certain drugs and equipment for emergency use and all technicians must know where they are kept. Some suggested items are the following:

Sterile syringes and needles for the administration of hypodermic, intravenous, or intramuscular medications
Aromatic spirits of ammonia for fainting

Ampules of Adrenalin to be used for allergic dye reactions, to raise blood pressure, and as a
  stimulant
Insulin for use in diabetic coma
50% glucose or sugar for insulin shock
Nitroglycerin for use in some types of cardiac pain
Amyl nitrate and caffeine as stimulants
Tourniquet
Blood pressure apparatus and stethoscope
Oxygen tank with mask
Electric suction apparatus
Airway
Laryngoscope

Provision of a well-equipped emergency box, and emergency supplies, and
the technician's knowledge of the *whereabouts* of the equipment can often save
a life in the department. Thinking through possible emergency situations is wise,
so that when immediate patient care *is* necessary, the technician does not panic,
but offers herself as a competent, steady, and dependable medical team member.

REFERENCES

Physical assistance in patient care

1. Brownell, K. O.: A textbook of practical nursing, ed. 4, Philadelphia, 1954, W. B. Saunders Co., chap. 9.
2. Dakin, F., and Thompson, E.: Simplified nursing, ed. 7, Philadelphia, 1960, J. B. Lippincott Co., 576-586.
3. Fash, B.: Body mechanics in nursing arts, New York, 1946, McGraw-Hill Book Co., Inc.
4. Goulding, F. A., and Torrop, H. M.: The practical nurse and her patient, Philadelphia, 1955, J. P. Lippincott Co., chap. 6.
5. Harmer, B., and Henderson, V.: Textbook of the principles and practice of nursing, New York, 1955, The Macmillan Co., chap. 15.
6. Howorth, M. B.: Dynamic posture, Hygeia **25**:198, 1947.
7. Howorth, M. B.: Posture in adolescents and adults, Amer. J. Nurs. **56**:34-36, 1956.
8. Mallory, E. F.: Immobilization—why and how, X-ray Technician **23**:17, 1951.
9. McClain, E. M., and Gragg, S. H.: Scientific principles in nursing, ed. 5, St. Louis, 1966, The C. V. Mosby Co.
10. Montag, M. L., and Swenson, R. P. S.; Fundamentals in nursing care, ed. 3, Philadelphia, 1959, W. B. Saunders Co., chap. 7.
11. Newton, K.: Preventing backstrain in nursing, Amer. J. Nurs. **43**:921, 1943.
12. Stevenson, J. L.: Posture and nursing, Joint Orthopedic Nursing Advisory Service of the NOPHN and NLNE, New York, 1948.
13. Wright, J.: Protective body mechanics in convalescence, Amer. J. Nurs. **45**:699, 1945.

Patient care affected by age and degree of consciousness

14. Brownell, K. O.: A textbook of practical nursing, ed. 4, Philadelphia, 1954, W. B. Saunders Co., chaps. 16, 17.
15. Charles, D. C.: Outstanding characteristics of older patients, Amer. J. Nurs. **61**:81-84, 1961.
16. Colwell, C.: Care of the geriatric patient, Nurs. Times **50**:890-892, 1954.
17. Dakin, F., and Thompson, E.: Simplified nursing, ed. 7, Philadelphia, 1960, J. B. Lippincott Co., chaps. 23, 25.
18. Emerson, C. P., Jr., and Bragdon, J. S.: Essentials of medicine, ed. 17, Philadelphia, 1955, J. B. Lippincott Co., chap. 7.
19. Faddis, M. O., and Hayman, J. M.: Care of the medical patient, New York, 1952, McGraw-Hill Book Co., Inc., chaps. 10, 11.

20. Flinauer, V., and Wallace, M.: Understanding a sick child's behavior, Amer. J. Nurs. **48**:517, 1948.
21. Frank, H.: Frightened child, Amer. J. Nurs. **51**:326-328, 1951.
22. Goulding, F. A., and Torrop, H. M.: The practical nurse and her patient, Philadelphia, 1955, J. B. Lippincott Co., chap. 20.
23. Hull, E., and Perrodin, C.: Medical nursing, ed. 4, Philadelphia, 1952, F. A. Davis Co., chap. 8.
24. Langford, W. S.: Physical illness and convalescence—their meaning to the child, J. Pediat. **33**:243-250, 1948.
25. Latham, N. C.: Safe care for hospitalized children, Amer. J. Nurs. **51**:403-404, 1951.
26. Lawton, G.: Aging successfully, New York, 1946, Columbia University Press.
27. Lyon, R. A., and Wallinger, E. M.: Mitchell's pediatrics and pediatric nursing, Philadelphia, 1950, W. B. Saunders Co., unit 4.
28. Merrill, A. P.: Special problems of the aged and the chronically ill, Hospitals **26**:61, 1952.
29. Montag, M. L., and Swenson, R. P. S.: Fundamentals in nursing care, ed. 3, Philadelphia, 1959, W. B. Saunders Co., chap. 26.
30. Newton, K.: Geriatric nursing, ed. 4, St. Louis, 1966, The C. V. Mosby Co., chap. 2.
31. Provost, L.: Pediatric x-ray—a formidable task?, X-ray Technician **33**:387-392, 1962.
32. Redel, F.: Understanding children's behavior, New York, 1950, Bureau of Publications, Teachers College, Columbia University.
33. Rudd, T. N.: The nursing of the elderly sick, Philadelphia, 1954, J. B. Lippincott Co.
34. Simpson, M. M.: The child in the hospital, Nurs. Times **48**:269, 1952.
35. Soffer, M. S.: Reducing anxiety in hospitalized children, Health News **31**:16-19, 1954.
36. X-ray procedure used in a children's hospital, Hosp. Manage. **73**:152-155, 1952.

First aid care of the patient in emergencies

37. American Red Cross first aid textbook, ed. 4, Philadelphia, 1957, Doubleday and Co.
38. Brownell, K. O.: A textbook of practical nursing, Philadelphia, 1954, W. B. Saunders Co., chap. 20.
39. Cecil, R., and Loeb, R.: A textbook of medicine, Philadelphia, 1955, W. B. Saunders Co., pp. 482-485.
40. Dakin, F., and Thompson, E.: Simplified nursing, ed. 7, Philadelphia, 1960, J. B. Lippincott Co., chap. 51.
41. Emerson, C. P., Jr., and Bragdon, J. S.: Essentials of medicine, ed. 17, Philadelphia, 1955, J. B. Lippincott Co., chap. 19.
42. Goulding, F. A., and Torrop, H. M.: The practical nurse and her patient, Philadelphia, 1955, J. B. Lippincott Co., chaps. 26 and 27.
43. Harmer, B., and Henderson, V.: Textbook of the principles and practice of nursing, New York, 1955, The Macmillan Co., chap. 43.
44. Hull, E., and Perrodin, C.: Medical nursing, ed. 4, Philadelphia, 1952, F. A. Davis Co., chap. 49.
45. Jensen, J., and Jensen, D. M.: Nursing in clinical medicine, New York, 1950, The Macmillan Co., unit 10.
46. Klein, H.: Nursing the allergic patient, Amer. J. Nurs. **46**:14-19, 1938.
47. Lennox, W. C.: The epileptic patient and the nurse, Amer. J. Nurs. **46**:219-233, 1946.
48. Maureen, Sister M., and Beland, I.: The nurse and the diabetic patient, Amer. J. Nurs. **46**:606-609, 1946.
49. Pennington, E.: Allergy and the allergic patient, Amer. J. Nurs. **38**:9-14, 1938.
50. Philberta, Sister M.: X-rays in emergencies, X-ray Technician **25**:36, 1953.
51. Rackemann, F. M.: The nurse and the patient with asthma, Amer. J. Nurs. **47**:463-566, 1947.
52. Stafford, E., and Dillar, D.: A textbook of surgery for nurses, Philadelphia, 1954, W. B. Saunders Co., chap. 6.
53. What not to do in caring for emergencies (editorial). Hosp. Prog. **35**:43-44, 1954.
54. Wooders, M. A., and Curtis, D. A.: Emergency care, Philadelphia, 1942, F. A. Davis Co., unit 1.

Chapter 4

Radiography and fluoroscopy—its hazards and special procedures

CONTRAST IN RADIOGRAPHY
General considerations

Rigler states that:

> . . . the x-ray film taken of any part of the body is simply a record of different densities. It is similar to a photographic film except that the source of light is an x-ray tube instead of ordinary lighting apparatus, and the "color" of the film depends upon the differences in density of the object photographed rather than upon differences in color. The denser or the thicker the object, the more rays will be absorbed by it and the less the exposure will be in that part of the film covered by it. The amount of radiation which reaches the film determines the amount of exposure, which is expressed in the film in terms of black and white. The less the exposure, or the less the amount of x-rays reaching the film, or the denser or thicker the part covering the film, the whiter will be that portion of the film. The exact reverse is also true. The x-ray film is therefore not simply a picture; it requires interpretation into terms of ordinary vision before it can be put to any use in diagnosis. The greater the skill in interpretation the more value the film will have in diagnosis. The technic of making the film is also of importance, but this is a comparatively simple matter. The interpretation depends upon a thorough knowledge of normal and pathological anatomy, of physiology, of clinical medicine, and of the various confusing factors of error which enter into the production of every x-ray film.*

In order to see the shadow of an organ it must lie next to another object of greater or lesser density than itself. Otherwise there will be no contrast between it and its surroundings and it cannot be distinguished as a separate organ. Thus, the humerus can be seen distinct from the muscles which surround it because of its greater density. The muscles usually cannot be distinguished from each other because their densities are approximately the same. If *natural* contrast is not present, *artificial* contrast is produced by the use of contrast media.

The shadows seen in the body and their distribution in order of their density, beginning with the lowest, are as follows:

Gas (air, oxygen)

    Normal distribution—in the sinuses, pharynx, the respiratory and gastrointestinal tract

---

*Rigler, L. G.: Outline of roentgen diagnosis, Atlas Edition, Philadelphia, 1938, J. B. Lippincott Co., p. 2.

Abnormal presence—either by injection of it into the brain, spinal canal, pleural cavity, or by pathologic condition such as obstruction, emphysema, and pneumothorax

Fat

Internal organs

Muscles

Blood-containing organs—the heart, blood vessels, liver

Calcium

Normal distribution—in the bones and organs

Abnormal presence—in tuberculous lesions in the lungs, valves of the heart, in the biliary tract or urinary tract

Foreign bodies—especially metallic, anywhere in the body

CONTRAST MEDIA
Types and qualities of contrast media

In the case of certain parts of the body, proper visualization is impossible because of the lack of natural contrast with the surrounding tissues. In order to overcome this handicap certain substances are used in various organs to produce this contrast, either by decreasing their density as, for example, by the introduction of a gas; or by increasing the density by the introduction of a heavy metallic salt.*

These substances are as follows:

Air or other gases—oxygen, carbon dioxide, used in pneumoencephalography

Heavy metallic salt—barium sulfate, used in gastrointestinal studies

Inorganic iodides—sodium, potassium, silver iodides, used for retrograde studies

Organic iodides—Priodax, Telepaque, Diodrast, Neo-Iopax, Cholografin, Urokon Sodium, Renografin, Miokin, Hypaque, Skiodan, Salpix, Dionosil, used for cholecystograms, angiograms (these are less irritating than some of the other contrast media)

Iodized oils (nonabsorbable)—Lipiodol, Iodochlorol

Iodized oils (slowly absorbable)—Pantopaque, Dionosil, used in bronchography

Contrast media must possess several qualities. They must show the structure clearly, creating a marked contrast with the density of surrounding tissues, and yet remain physiologically inert, that is, not permanently alter the appearance of the organ or area or affect its function. They must produce as little toxicity as possible to the patient, and they must be eliminated unchanged.

Preparation and administration

These contrast media are prepared and administered in a variety of ways. In examination of the gastrointestinal tract, for example, the contrast medium

---

*Rigler, L. G.: Outline of Roentgen diagnosis, Atlas Edition, Philadelphia, 1938, J. B. Lippincott Co., pp. 6-8.

is given orally or rectally, not intravenously. Barium sulfate, being a heavy metallic salt, offers good contrast to the hollow organs of the gastrointestinal tract. It is nontoxic, although it may cause constipation if not evacuated. Oral dyes can be prepared in either tablet or capsule form or powder form, as barium sulfate.

For examination of the urinary tract, as a further example, the contrast medium must be administered either directly into the urinary tract or indirectly into the blood stream, then excreted by and visualized in the urinary tract. Both the circulatory and excretory systems are sterile areas, and contrast media are prepared in vials or ampules.

A vial is a small bottle with a rubber stopper containing several doses. The medium must be withdrawn, using sterile technique, with a needle and syringe. An ampule is a vacuum-sealed container which generally has just enough solution for a single dose. It is opened by filing and snapping off its top. Here again, sterile technique and a needle and syringe are used in its administration.

In most hospitals the technicians give only barium and oral dyes because of their limited knowledge of sterile technique, pharmacology, and general medicine and because of the potential danger in administering the other media. The radiologist should be the one to select, draw into the syringe, and administer the intravenous types of material.

The handling of opaque media must always be considered seriously. Regardless of how long the technician has used them, deliberate care and caution must be taken in their selection and administration to the patient. Since the patient's safety and welfare are of prime importance, the following rules must be observed when using contrast media:

1. Be sure you have the *right patient* by asking him his name and checking carefully the name on the chart.

2. Be sure you have the *right contrast medium* and the *right amount*. Check the label three times—when you select it, when you pour it, and when you put it back on the shelf.

3. Be sure you give the contrast medium at the *right time*—when the radiologist specifically orders it so that its concentration is at its peak at the correct time.

4. Never handle a tablet or powder with your fingers. Pour the proper number of tablets into the cover of the bottle and then into a paper container or medicine glass, not your hand.

5. Record, in the proper places on the patient's chart, the amount of medium given, the time, and your initials.

Sensitivity

Many patients are sensitive in varying degrees to the iodine compounds. Local reactions at the site of administration can be pain, burning and itching, or numbness. But the patient may also have a generalized body reaction. The symptoms of sensitivity may be flushing of the face with increased salivation, increased tearing and nasal secretion, itching, hives, choking or asthma, nausea and vomiting, pallor, fainting, chills, or a state of shock.

The technician and the radiologist always ask the patient before an iodine dye is administered whether he has ever had or reacted to it before or if he has a history of allergy. If any sensitivity is suspected or if the patient has ever had hay fever, asthma, or hives, a special test is usually carried out. A drop of a dilute solution of the dye is placed either on the tongue or conjunctival sac in the eye. If the patient is sensitive to the dye, there will be marked redness, itching, and general irritation in 10 to 15 minutes. An antihistimine may be administered and the examination continued. Or the examination may be cancelled and an alternative one attempted.

When a patient must undergo an examination involving a contrast medium that produces ill effects, the technician should always tell him what to expect— that he may feel flushed, that he may be a little nauseated, or that he may have a choking sensation. It is wise for the technician to be on guard at all times during the procedure for a more severe reaction; he should watch the patient closely. Allergic persons are somewhat more likely to have untoward reactions to contrast agents and should be watched particularly closely. Knowledge of the emergency drug box, its contents, and whereabouts are essential. The radiologist may wish to administer Adrenalin to slow the absorption or alter the effect of the contrast medium. Or he may wish to administer certain other medications to the distressed patient.

FLUOROSCOPY
General considerations

Fluoroscopy is a process which permits the studying of internal structures *at a given time,* by the use of an x-ray machine consisting of an x-ray transformer and control, an x-ray tube, and a special fluorescent screen. It is not a permanent record like a radiograph but rather enables the radiologist to view an area directly.

Most fluoroscopic screens are relatively inefficient, giving poor contrast between light and dark shadows. Therefore, in order to best compare the contrast of these black and white shadows several things are done. First, fluoroscopy is carried on in nearly total darkness, thereby reducing extraneous light distractions in the periphery of the examining room and making the shadow contrast maximal on the fluoroscopic screen. Second, the radiologist wears red goggles for a period of 15 to 30 minutes before he begins the fluoroscopic examination in order to dark adapt his eyes, making them more able to discern shadow variations. The red goggles enable a part of the retina which functions best in dim light to take over. Third, barium sulfate is frequently given as the contrast medium, and being opaque, it casts definite shadows on the area to be examined, again increasing shadow contrast and making easier diagnosis between the center or lumen of hollow body organs being examined and their soft tissue walls.

Dark adaptation

Probably everyone has had the experience of going to a matinee and can recall that in leaving the bright sunshine and entering the theater there was great difficulty in seeing. Despite the help of an usher, one usually stumbles over people already seated, has difficulty in finding the arms of the chair, and is unaware of whether someone is seated adjacently. After a short time, vision improves. This is due to a fairly rapid process called accommodation and a slower process called dark adaptation. Both processes are essential to proper diagnosis and patient care during fluoroscopic procedures.

Accommodation of the eye, or altering the focus so that light rays are brought together on the retina, is accomplished by action of the lens. This *lens* accommodation plus *pupil* contraction occurs almost instantly upon leaving a bright area and entering a dark area, or vice versa. However, dark adaptation which is the adjustment of the *retina* in raising its threshold of sensitivity to light, takes from fifteen minutes to one-half hour. The radiologist dark adapts by wearing red goggles and can move freely about the x-ray department readying himself for fluoroscopy. The technician, however, in order to best assist the radiologist and the patient, dark adapts by remaining in the dark fluoroscopic room the necessary time.

Fluoroscopy with the image intensifier

The previous paragraphs have described conventional fluoroscopy and the importance of eye adaption. The retina of the eye has a layer of structures which are called rod and cone structures. When an eye is dark adapted, most of the vision available is made possible by the rods in this structure. If there is an abundance of light present, however, the biggest share of the vision is made available through the cone structures. To simplify, the rod structures have a facility for picking up dimly lit objects but with a poor ability to resolve the details of the objects. The cone structures, on the other hand, when sufficient light is available, do have the ability to resolve the details of an object well. Dark adaption, therefore, generates rod vision in the eye and submerges cone vision. A device that has radically changed the approach to fluoroscopy is the image intensifier. An image intensifier can take the dimly lit fluoroscopic image and electronically increase its brilliance many thousand times. The image intensifier has added new dimensions to fluoroscopy. These are as follows:

1. The radiologist, when viewing the fluoroscopic image with an image intensifier, is using his cone vision and, therefore, is revolving more details than he could when viewing with rod vision inherent in conventional fluoroscopy.

2. As this electronic image is many thousand times more brilliant than the

fluoroscopic image without any increase in the radiation dose to the patient, it is now safe to make motion picture studies of the fluoroscopic image.

3. The use of television camera and closed-circuit television is also made possible by the increased brightness of the image, and in this instance, viewing is accomplished by using a television monitor similar to your television set at home. It is therefore possible to have what might be called "conference" or "teaching" fluoroscopy because more than one person can view the image with the radiologist in charge of the case.

4. The possibility of tape recording the televised image becomes possible.

5. Image-intensified fluoroscopy radically aids in care and comfort of the patient.

With this system it is not necessary to have a completely darkened room; the patient, if he is ambulatory, can move freely and follow directions more easily; the fear of being in the dark, which is common with patients, particularly children, is eliminated, and if the examination is of a type that requires parallel procedures, for example, the insertion of a catheter or the injection of a contrast medium, it is facilitated by the fact that the patient knows what is going on, and the people concerned with the patient's examination do have ordinary light to use without interferring with the fluoroscopic image.

An interesting phenomenon occurs in x-ray departments where there is a mixture of fluoroscopic equipment, some of the conventional type and some with image intensifiers. If the radiologist is alternating examinations between an image-intensifier fluoroscopic room and a conventional fluoroscopic room, as the day procedes the image-intensifier room will apparently become less efficient. The image will become more brilliant, but the ability to perceive detail will become less on the part of the radiologist. The reason is that the radiologist, as he fluoroscopes in the conventional room, will start to become dark adapted, and when he returns to the image-intensifier room, his rod vision will be perceiving the image rather than his cone vision. It follows, therefore, that technologists and radiologists should not become dark adapted if they are using an image intensifier.

RADIATION HAZARD
Protection of the patient and medical team

An extremely important aspect of patient care in x-ray technology, and a responsibility shared by the radiologist and the technician, is safeguarding the patient and medical team from overexposure to radiation. The medical profession and its technical associates have long recognized that overexposure to various types of radiant energy, including that emitted by an x-ray tube, are hazardous to health. This hazard involves not only the person receiving the radiation but also those persons responsible for the operation of the sources emitting the radiation as well as anyone else in the area who is unprotected. It has been shown that repeated exposure to x-rays is harmful to the reproductive system, can cause increased incidence of sterility, or can have serious effect on future offspring of the person exposed. Moreover, radiation overexposure may cause bone marrow disease or tissue destruction. It is not too uncommon even these days to see an elderly physician with scarred hands, a result of x-ray burns received when the science was young and the dangers of overexposure were unknown. Technicians are fortunate to have working for their welfare a Committee on X-ray Protection as part of the American Society of Radiologic Technologists. It is the responsibility of the technicians to protect themselves and to follow all the Committee's suggestions and regulations for their safety.

As students in x-ray technology, most technicians have received adequate training in protection of themselves and their associates from radiation exposure. This includes wearing leaded aprons during fluoroscopy and stepping into control booths during the taking of films. In most departments personnel wear an x-ray–sensitive film badge that indicates the amount of radiation to which they have been exposed in a given period. Technicians can then limit their exposure to within safe limits in a given period. Radiologists wear leaded gloves during fluoroscopy, since their hands come into direct exposure with the radiation.

On the other hand, most technicians have *not* had sufficient instruction in their responsibilities toward protecting the *patient* from radiation hazards in medical diagnosis and treatment. They do know such hazards exist, but they are unaware of what they personally can do to assist in limiting radiation to a patient.

Recent increased emphasis

This problem has become *more* acute due to our arrival at the atomic age and the effect of the latter on increase of background radiation to which all people are exposed. In June, 1957, the National Academy of Sciences, including a committee of atomic physicists, geneticists, and radiation specialists, released a report giving information on radiation to the general population of the world. It aroused considerable medical and lay interest and discussion concerning the use of medical x-rays. With increasing use of radiation in the Armed Forces, in industry, and in medicine, technicians must enlarge their understanding of the whole problem and realize the magnitude of *their* role in cutting down radiation exposure to the patient to within the limits of patient safety.

Knowledge of technical terms and radiation dosimetry is essential. The technician may not use these terms in day-to-day technical work, but careful, skilled technicians who read the technical literature and keep abreast of their profession will find an understanding of terminology helpful and necessary. An understanding is also necessary of those persons in allied technical fields who share this concern for the patient and the general public.

roentgen a unit of X or gamma radiation.

milli- represents one one-thousandth of any unit it prefixes. Therefore, a milliroentgen is one one-thousandth of a roentgen.

rep the energy absorption dose in a radiated tissue of 93 ergs per gram.

rad the energy absorption dose of 100 ergs per gram and a simpler method to describe energy absorption dose.

genetics a branch of biology which deals with the phenomenon of heredity and variation. It seeks to understand the causes of resemblances and differences between parents and their progeny.

mutation a change of form of variable extent from that normally passed on from one generation to another. Some are good, most are detrimental to life of the offspring, and all are unpredictable. Mutations come about by some alteration of the egg or sperm or by abnormal amounts of radiation.

health physics a branch of radiological physics dealing with the protection of personnel and patients from harmful effects of ionizing radiation.

primary radiation the emission and propagation of energy through space.

secondary radiation that resulting from the interaction of primary radiation with matter.

background radiation that which results from natural causes, such as cosmic rays, naturally occurring radium, to which all people are exposed.

Geneticists say that in order to avoid undesirable mutations in future generations, the *maximum permissible* dose for the average population to receive from conception to the age of 30 is 10 roentgens. To emphasize the gravity of the situation even further, the International Committee on Radiological Protection calls this the *minimum possible* dose. They estimate that background radiation alone will contribute 3 roentgens of radiation to the gonads or reproductive organs by the age of 30, *exclusive* of any medical or artificial radiation. The accuracy of these figures is not firmly established, since the understanding of radiation and its effects is in an evolutionary stage. However, all qualified people, including physicians and geneticists, agree that the danger does exist and that the population must be safeguarded. The United States Atomic Energy Commission is constantly carrying on research as is the International Committee on Radiological Protection. The way in which this dose is determined or whether it could be exceeded when medical judgment dictates is not the responsibility of the technician. However, it *is* the concern and responsibility of the technician to keep the radiation to the patient at an absolute minimum necessary to produce results which will aid in his diagnosis and treatment. Also, radiologists must always balance the need for a patient's x-ray procedure against the risk or radiation hazard involved.

Methods of limiting overexposure

The technician can limit overexposure by use of proper filtration, cones, diaphragms, lead rubber or lead cloth, and proper darkroom technique and exposure factors.

Proper filtration. For many years it had been the custom of x-ray manufacturers to supply their x-ray equipment with 0.5 mm. aluminum as a filter in the tube aperture. This was considered adequate to filter out nonuseful long wave lengths. It is now recommended by the Bureau of Standards of the United States Government that the filtration in radiographic tubes be increased to 2.5 mm. of aluminum. It was determined that while this amount has no effect on the exposure factors and general technique, except in the lower kilovoltage range, it *does* allow for a marked decrease, up to 15 to 20%, in the skin and the gonadal dose to the patient. On this basis, therefore, during the average antero-posterior view of a skull, using only 0.5 mm. of aluminum as a filter, the skin dose to the skull would be 800 to 1,000 milliroentgens. The gonadal dose would be approximately 3.85 milliroentgens, received in the form of secondary radiation from the primarily exposed portion of the anatomy, in this instance, the skull. The technician must remember that regardless of the part of the body being radiographed there is always a secondary radiation dose to the gonads. The simple addition of 2 mm. more of aluminum to the tube aperture would cut down the skin dose to 600 milliroentgens on an anteroposterior skull and also decrease the gonadal dose to the patient.

As further evidence, assuming that only 0.5 mm. of filtration is used, the average radiograph of a lateral lumbar spine requires approximately 3,500 milliroentgens of exposure. This results in the male receiving a dose of 70 milliroentgens to the gonads and the female a dose of 350 milliroentgens. This difference in gonadal dose is due to the difference in anatomic location of gonads in the male and the female. The addition of 2 mm. of aluminum however, and without a change in exposure factors, would reduce the skin dose to 2,300 milliroentgens, the gonadal dose to the male to 40 milliroentgens and the gonadal dose to the female to 240 milliroentgens. Therefore, it is obvious that the simple addition of aluminum plates will universally reduce both the skin dose and the gonadal dose to a marked degree. This is particularly true in exposures involving the gonadal area, such as radiography and fluoroscopy of the abdomen, colon, spine, and pelvis. Therefore, it becomes the technician's responsibility personally to examine the aperture of the x-ray tubes in use in their departments to ensure that proper filtration is present.

Cones, collimators, and diaphragms. The proper use of collimation is another factor in decreasing the radiation hazard. For example, using correct filtration and careful collimation in radiographing a skull will decrease the skin dose to the skull but also will markedly decrease the gonadal dose to the patient. When a cone is not used by the technician, the skin dose to the patient is increased twice as much and covers a much wider area of the body. The gonadal dose is about six to eight times as much when a cone is not used. This is due to the fact that *some* of the divergent *primary* radiation reaches toward that portion of the anatomy where the gonads are located. Therefore, the technician, in order to exercise proper precautions against over-radiation must always use a cone, preferably a triple diaphragm cone. It must be arranged to cover only the part that is to be radiographed, thereby limiting the divergent beams which might radiate to other portions of the patient's anatomy without having any desirable effect on the radiograph. Fortunately the use of cones and diaphragms by the technician can only improve films by limiting the amount of secondary radiation which is hitting the x-ray film during the course of the exposure. Some technicians hesitate to cone parts sharply, fearing that the radiograph will not include a wide enough area. True, while making an x-ray exposure technicians must think of the quality of the film they are producing and whether or not the designated anatomic portion will appear on the film. But on the other hand, they must also remember that any error in coning has a marked effect on the gonadal dose to the patient.

Lead cloth and rubber. The use of lead cloth or lead rubber in x-ray departments has unfortunately been widely disregarded. As an example, the film files of many well-regarded institutions show the abdomen as well as the chest on the film in nearly all of the infant chest exposures. In these cases, then, the technician has been guilty of giving a markedly increased gonadal dose to the patient without its serving any useful purpose as far as the medical diagnosis is concerned, and this at a time when the patient is most susceptible to radiation. In an infant chest x-ray exposures, if triple diaphragm cones are used properly, the gonadal dose is limited markedly. The addition of a piece of lead cloth or lead rubber over the abdomen of the infant, leaving only the chest unprotected, results in far greater protection to the infant.

It was stated previously that the permissible gonadal dose was 10 roentgens from conception to age 30. Therefore, the protection of the pregnant woman is a special x-ray problem where radiation hazard is concerned. Medical judgment will often dictate that certain examinations be done on the pregnant woman. But in all cases where the abdomen is not concerned in the examination, it should be covered with lead cloth or lead rubber to minimize the gonadal dose not only to the pregnant woman herself but also to the infant in the uterus. Susceptibility to radiation is much more pronounced in the unborn child. This is a precaution that must be observed.

Darkroom technique and proper exposure factors. The use of proper darkroom technique and proper exposure factors is one of the best tools a technician has in limiting undesirable, useless radiation to a patient. Carelessness or lack of proper procedure by the technician often results in "re-dos" or repeat films. And in each instance where a repeat film is necessary there is a double dose to the gonads and skin of the patient. A primary factor in preventing unnecessary radiation to the patients lies within the technician's desire to become an expert and a responsible person, concerned in carrying out his work. It is impossible to limit *all* "re-dos" in x-ray technology. But those that are not the fault of poor preparation, movement, or equipment breakdown should be limited. One of the most important aims of all technicians should be to avoid unnecessary exposure of a patient due to carelessness. Some typical examples of carelessness are cited. A technique may call for *100* milliamperes at *75* KVP on the *small* focal spot for one patient. On the succeeding patient, it may call for *300* Ma. at *75* or *80* KVP on the large focal spot. Due to carelessness the technician may not change the monitor from *100* to *300* between patients and may realize this fact only after exposure. In most x-ray departments a repeat film is the result, but a hidden result is the double dose to the gonads and skin of that patient for this one examination.

A technician may neglect to place a lead "L" or "R" marker on the film and realize it only when the film is processed. The technician has two choices. The first is to retake the film and double the gonadal dose to the patient. Or second, and the method of choice, the technician can turn in the film, report the error and together with the radiologist, determine which side is "L" and which is "R." It will take time, it may irritate the radiologist, and it may result in personal criticism. But the technician with integrity and concern for the patient's safety will attempt to use the film with the error as the diagnostic film in the case and take the personal consequences. When it becomes a choice between personal criticism in the department and unnecessary radiation to the patient, a technician should use good judgment, admit the error, and allow the radiologist, not the technician, to decide whether the need for a repeat film is present. In this section the gonadal dose has been emphasized because of its prime importance. However, in limiting the gonadal dose one also limits skin dose. Unnecessary radiation to the patient and *all* medical team members in the room is also limited.

Alternative methods of limiting radiation

There are other ways of decreasing radiation exposure to the patient. These methods *do* have some effect on film quality, however, which the four previously mentioned do not. Therefore, it rests with the radiologist's judgment whether to compromise on film quality in order to lessen the radiation dose to the patient, or whether the need for better film quality will contribute to the diagnosis to such a degree that it outweighs the increased radiation hazard to the patient. There are available several different speeds of film, different speed screens, and nonscreen film. The use of the various radiographic accessories results in increasing or decreasing the exposure time, depending upon the accessory or film being used. Ideally there will be less exposure to the patient and therefore a decreased gonadal dose if high speed screens with high speed film are used. Unfortunately this results in some screen grain, possibly interfering with the diagnosis due to lack of detail. For this reason the technician must consult the radiologist when these accessories are used. However, high speed screens and high speed film should be available in every department and should certainly be considered whenever x-raying a pregnant woman or on all patients where long heavy exposures are necessary. Although the quality of the film might not appeal to the radiologist with the artistic eye, it nevertheless will have sufficient information to make the proper diagnosis, thereby ensuring the proper medical treatment for the patient without increasing his gonadal or skin dose which would be inherent in using a finer detail accessory or film.

STERILE TECHNIQUE
Contrast between medical and surgical asepsis

In order to be a skillful assistant and to give the best possible care to the patient, the technician must have an understanding of sterile technique and must be aware of the precautions in handling equipment and supplies that will be used in certain diagnostic x-ray procedures. This is discussed here because most contrast media need to be administered with a needle and syringe *using* sterile technique. In preceding chapters the use of medical asepsis has been discussed—some of the methods used to prevent the spread of bacteria from a contaminated center *outward*. In ordinary handwashing, for example, the aim is to prevent bacteria and contamination on the technician's hands from being carried *to* patients, x-ray tables, linen, and other articles. In gowning for infant care, the aim is to prevent any soil or bacteria on the technician's uniform from leaving that contaminated center and spreading outward, contaminating the baby. In the following chapter the technician will learn that in gowning and scrubbing for portable radiography for an isolated patient, again the aim is to keep the contamination localized and prevent it from spreading and being carried elsewhere by the technician's hands, uniform, or machine.

In surgical asepsis, however, the aim is to prevent the entry of bacteria *into* a *sterile* area. The technique used to effect this is called sterile technique. Sterile technique need not be used for gastrointestinal radiography since the gastrointestinal tract is not a sterile area. For example, we do not eat sterile food. However, sterile technique *is* necessary when there is introduction of any instrument or needle into sterile body cavities such as the urinary tract, the central nervous system, or the circulatory system. Sterilization of supplies used is necessary in order to kill not only disease-producing bacteria but also all other bacteria.

A suggested procedure

The aim of surgical asepsis, in any procedure where it is required, is to keep bacteria that are everywhere in the x-ray room—on the tables, machines, and technician's hands—from coming in contact with any material or supplies that will be used during the procedure and thereby from entering the patient, increasing the chance for infection in the area being examined. Although the technician may not touch a needle which will be used to introduce the contrast medium, the needle could become contaminated by having it touch a part of the tray that the technician has brushed against and *become unsterile.*

A suggested procedure for maintaining surgical asepsis follows:

1. Wash the hands well for general cleanliness.

2. Gloves for the doctor should be opened carefully with the wrapper held open and should not be allowed to snap back to contaminate the gloves. They should be opened with the fingers pointing toward the technician and the wrist or opened end toward the doctor. Sizes 7 and 7½ generally fit the doctor; the sizes are marked on the outside of the glove packages (Fig. 4-1).

3. Place the tray with sterile contents on an instrument stand or table which will be large enough and conveniently close to the doctor's working area.

4. In opening the tray, remove the string or adhesive and unwrap it in such

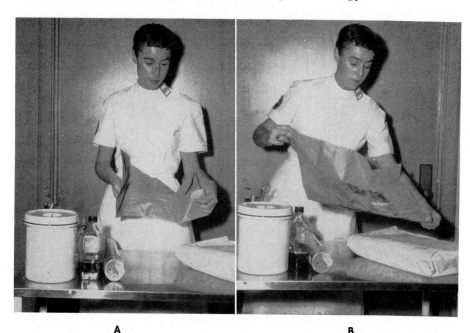

A	**B**

Fig. 4-1. Opening a glove package. The technician opens the glove package for the doctor, holding the package at the edge and in such a fashion that the wrists of the gloves are toward him.

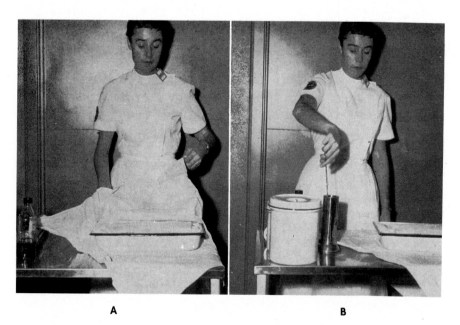

A	**B**

Fig. 4-2. Sterile technique. **A,** The technician opens a pneumoencephalogram tray whose contents are sterile. She is careful not to pass her arm over the tray. **B,** The forceps are lifted directly out of the container, not tapped at the edge.

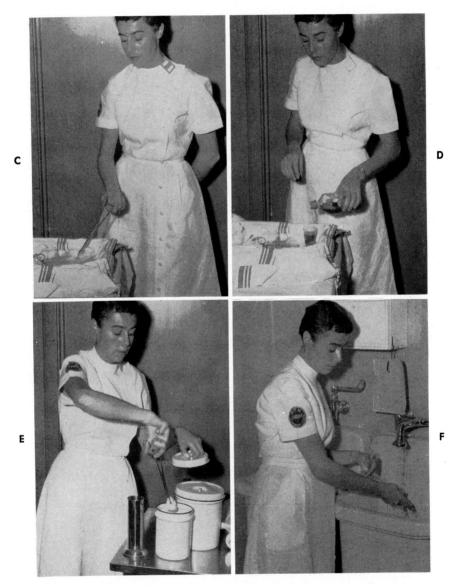

Fig. 4-2, cont'd. C, The tray contents are set into position, placing medicine glasses to one side but leaving an arbitrary inch around as unsterile. The technician's other arm is out of the way of the sterile field. **D,** A solution is poured, keeping the label side of the bottle up. The bottle must not touch the sterile medicine glass. **E,** Cotton balls are lifted directly out of the sterile cannister with the cover held correctly. **F,** At the completion of a procedure, glassware, syringes, and needles are rinsed with cold water before placing them back on the tray to be sent to the central supply room.

a way that the arms do not pass over the opened tray and contaminate it. At all times, avoid bending over or passing equipment over the open tray (Fig. 4-2, *A*).

5. All the equipment inside the tray is sterile and must be handled by the doctor with sterile rubber gloves or by the technician with sterile forceps. Sterile equipment immediately becomes contaminated if anything unsterile touches it.

6. Forceps should be kept in quart jars or forcep jars and should be immersed *to the handles* in disinfectant solution. Instrument Zephiran, which is regular Zephiran with an antirust compound added, is often used. In removing forceps, lift them directly up. Do not tap them on the edge of the container, since the area not *in* Zephiran is not sterile. They must be held with the tips down at all times, not waved about or inverted, since the solution remaining on the forceps would run down, touch the unsterile portion of the forceps near the fingers, and when returned to position carry the bacteria back to the sterile part, thus contaminating it. If contamination does occur at any time, sterile forceps should be obtained for immediate use and the contaminated forceps should be boiled for 10 minutes. Simply reimmersing them in the disinfectant does not sterilize them—it merely disinfects them. Remember, disinfection does not kill *all* bacteria (Fig. 4-2, *B*).

7. An arbitrary area of 1 inch around each edge of the tray is considered unsterile as an extra safeguard.

8. With the forceps move the medicine glasses or basins on the tray to the edge, avoiding this outer inch, and set them upright (Fig. 4-2, *C*).

9. Return the forceps to the jar immediately after each use.

10. The two solutions necessary for these procedures are tincture of Zephiran or some other disinfectant to clean the injection site and Novocain to anesthetize the area. Tincture of Zephiran is regular Zephiran with 70% alcohol added. Carefully select each bottle. The caps should be held with the inner side down while pouring the solution. However, if it is necessary to lay the cap down, it should be placed with the inside uppermost to prevent any contamination of the inner surface. Hold the bottle, with the label up, in the palm of the hand, so that if any solution drips when pouring from the bottle it will not deface the label making it difficult to read (Fig. 4-2, *D*).

11. Pour the amount of solution desired by the doctor in the glass. Do not touch the sterile medicine glass with the unsterile solution bottle. If the bottle has a cap, not a cork, and the lip is protected, it is not necessary to pour a small amount of solution into a waste basin first. Care must be taken to avoid spilling on the tray, since moisture carries contamination and any wet area is considered unsterile. Other sterile equipment on the tray must not touch the wet area.

12. If a *vial* of Novocain is used instead of the bottle, select it from the shelf, hold the label so the doctor can see it, and grasp the vial firmly. The doctor, not touching the vial itself, will clean off its rubber stopper with a Zephiran-

soaked cotton ball, plunge the needle into the vial and withdraw the contents into his syringe while the technician holds the vial.

13. Any sterile equipment that the doctor asks for which may not be on the tray, such as cotton balls or gauze squares, should be obtained from sterile cannisters with sterile forceps. The covers of the containers should also be held with the inner side down while removing the contents (Fig. 4-2, *E*).

14. Sterile equipment once removed from a sterile cannister can never be replaced in the cannister at any time, even though it has not been used. Therefore, care should be taken to withdraw only the desired amount. Any unused sterile equipment can be labeled "clean" and sent down to the central supply room to be placed in cannisters and reautoclaved (Fig. 4-2, *F*).

15. When sterile cannisters are empty or if their contents become contaminated due to any break in sterile technique, their covers should be inverted. They should be labeled "unsterile" and returned to the central supply room for refilling and reautoclaving.

16. Once a week the solution in forceps jars should be discarded, the jars boiled for 10 minutes and refilled with fresh solution.

It is important that the technician understand that a procedure of this type is necessary to the safety of the patient. It is not just an arbitrary set of rules, hard to follow and complicating the technician's role. It must be further remembered that the usual patient is ill. Whereas a break in technique and resultant contamination of a sterile body cavity *may* have no ill effect on a well person, it may greatly complicate the condition of an ill patient. Foreign bacteria in the central nervous system can cause meningitis or encephalitis. Entry and growth in the urinary tract may cause pyelitis or cystitis. It is obvious that not *every* break in sterile technique results in illness, but it is the responsibility of all members of the medical team to use all possible precautions to prevent any contamination and thus preclude possible illness. If during a procedure the technician does contaminate something, wisdom and integrity would demand immediate reporting to the physician so that the piece of apparatus could be discarded. The technician should never refrain from prompt reporting of contamination for fear it will show up his ignorance or incompetence. The safety of the patient is of prime importance, and a team member who recognizes contamination when he sees it, reports it, and helps correct it is much more to be admired than one who uses careless technique with a flourish and demonstrates superficial competence.

A combination of various disposable products will be seen in the composition of disposable trays used in x-ray departments. For example, the lumbar puncture tray used in connection with a myelogram may be made up of disposable products. Sterile technique should not be decreased because of the use of disposable products. If strict sterile technique is maintained where it is required, the chance of infection should be lowered by using disposable products. It becomes the technician's responsibility not only to handle the disposable products in an approved fashion but also to examine the packaging. There are many ways that a packaged sterile product that has been prepared at the manufacturers could be contaminated by the time that it arrives in your department.

In the process of being transported from the manufacturer, the wholesaler, and then the hospital's supply area, the material could have been left standing on a loading dock, for example, during a heavy rain or snowstorm. If some of the packages had become moistened, they could have had a sealed edge loosened that later had resealed itself; but, of course, in this instance, the package would no longer be sterile.

Any sign of discoloration, fraying, or any other type of alteration in the configuration of the package should act as a warning signal to the technician to set that particular product aside.

It is probably wise and, in fact, a custom in most hospitals to send samples of sterile disposable products to their laboratories for evaluation from time to time. In the case of the tampered or altered package, the department using it should also send this package to the laboratories for checking.

Finally, the use of sterile disposable products and even the surgically clean disposable products creates a problem. This problem is what is to be done with these things after they are used. When using nondisposable sterile equipment, the usual procedure is to clean it, wash it, and prepare it for sterilization.

When using disposable products, it is not necessary and not even practical to sterilize the used products. It is necessary, however, to have an orderly system of discarding contaminated or used disposable equipment. This is not only necessary at the departmental level but is also a problem at the hospital level. The disposable products should not be left in the examining room area at the end of an examination, but rather taken to a central area in the department to be picked up and disposed of by the hospital in whatever manner has been evolved. Some examples of disposable products may be seen in Fig. 4-3.

HYPODERMIC INJECTION

The word "hypodermic" means pertaining to the region beneath the skin. Therefore, hypodermic injection would mean injection beneath the skin. If the injection is directly into a vein, it would properly be called an intravenous hypodermic injection; if into a muscle, an intramuscular hypodermic injection; and if into the skin, an intradermal hypodermic injection.

Normally, hypodermic injections are not within the range of the duties performed by radiologic technologists. However, one must be thoroughly familiar with the technique of preparation and administration of hypodermic injections.

Hazards and precautions in hypodermic injections

The administration of a drug hypodermically is far different from one given orally. The precautions for giving oral contrast media, for example, have already been mentioned. These same precautions must be recalled, emphasized, and

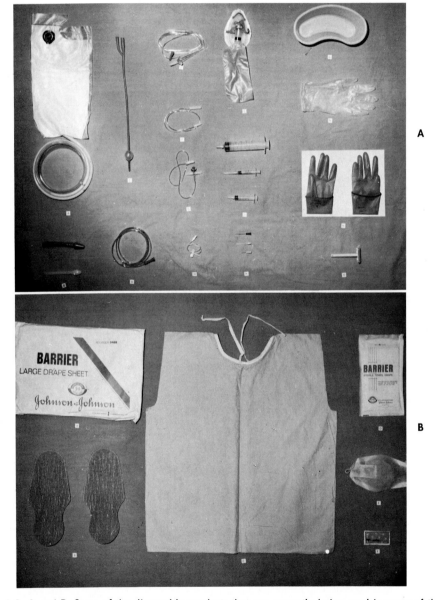

Fig. 4-3. A and **B,** Some of the disposable products that are currently being used in many of the departments of radiology.

effected in the administration of contrast media or medications which may be given hypodermically.

A material given hypodermically is absorbed by the blood stream much faster than one given orally. Consequently, its action is much faster, and therefore, its administration usually has more serious implications.

It is absolutely imperative to be sure of the four "rights." These are as follows: (1) The *right patient*. One must be sure that the patient is the person for whom the medication or contrast media has been prescribed. One must be sure that there are no contraindications for the material listed on the request for the x-ray procedure. (2) The *right drug or contrast medium*. It is vital to check the ampule or rubber-stoppered vial label several times to make sure that the material is the proper one. (3) The *right amount*. The amount ordered by the physician in charge should be checked, and only this amount should be given to the patient. (4) The *right time*—to ensure maximum visualization of the contrast medium. For example, the medium must be given at the time ordered to ensure proper visualization at the time the x-ray examination is being made.

Necessary equipment

Hypodermic syringes and needles are available in a variety of sizes and may be either the disposable type or the nondisposable type. Syringes are roughly classified by capacity in either milliliters or cubic centimeters.

Needles are said to be a certain gauge in size; the lumen (hole) is the basis of classification. The needle is further classified by length. For example, comparing a 19-gauge × 1½ needle with a 24-gauge × 1½ needle, we would find the 19-gauge needle would have a larger lumen than the 24-gauge needle, but they would both be 1½ inches in length.

A basic hypodermic injection tray in general use in x-ray departments is one used for the coventional intravenous pyelogram examination (see Fig. 4-4). It should include syringes and needles of proper size, a piece of rubber tubing to be used as a tourniquet, the selected contrast medium in an ampule or rubber-stoppered vial, and a bottle of disinfective solution such as alcohol or Zephiran. Also, a sterile cannister of cotton balls and a pair of forceps in a sterile solution should be available.

Techniques for withdrawing a contrast medium from ampule or rubber-stoppered vial

A suggested method is for the technician to procede as follows:

1. If a nondisposable syringe is used, the first step is to assemble the syringe and protect the sterility of the needle being applied to the syringe with a sterile gauze square.

2. If an ampule is used, it is necessary to have a small steel file.

3. In either instance, the next step is to withdraw a cotton ball from a sterile cannister.

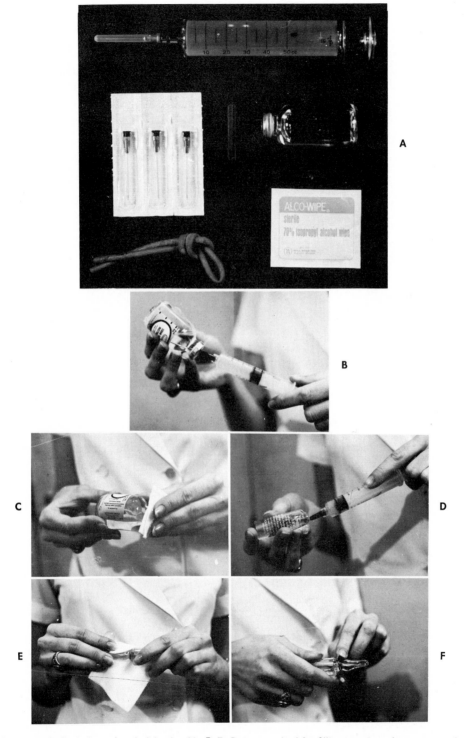

Fig. 4-4. A, Basic hypodermic injection kit. **B-F,** Proper method for filling a syringe from an ampule or a rubber-stoppered vial. The actual filling of the syringe follows injection of air through the syringe into the rubber-stoppered vial.

4. Moisten it with a disinfectant and thoroughly scrub the steel file and the ampule or the rubber-stoppered vial.

5. With the barrel of the syringe partially withdrawn, insert needle in the vial and close syringe to inject air into the vial about equal to the amount of contrast that is to be withdrawn.

6. Slowly withdraw the contents up into the syringe barrel by pulling on the top of the plunger, not its length, with the right hand.

7. If air enters the syringe, remove it from the ampule or rubber-stoppered vial and tilt the syringe up so that the needle is uppermost, and the air, being lighter than the syringe contents, will rise. Merely push the plunger up until the air is expelled.

8. After the correct amount of contrast is withdrawn pull back a bit on the plunger so that air comes into the syringe. Then in carrying it to the patient, if the plunger is moved at all, only air escapes and not the desired amount of the contrast medium.

9. Place the needle back on the sterile guaze square while you obtain a dry cotton ball with sterile forceps from a cannister. Place the cotton ball on the syringe using forceps; this ensures its sterility while carrying it to the patient.

10. Secure a second cotton ball, moisten it with the disinfectant. This is used to clean the injection site on the patient.

The syringe is now ready to hand to the doctor, who will make the actual injection. In any procedure involving a technique of this kind, the technician must not concentrate on the mechanics of the procedure to the extent that the patient and his feelings become secondary. Therefore, it is wise to be sure of all steps of the procedure and become adept in practice situations first. When the patient must receive the contrast medium, he is still the core of concern, not the special technique.

REFERENCES

1. Adams, R.: Prevention of infection in hospitals, Amer. J. Nurs. **58**:344, 1958.
2. Benson, M. E.: Handwashing—an important part of medical asepsis, Amer. J. Nurs. **57**:1136, 1957.
3. Collier, M. E.: Drugs and their administration, Nursing Mirror 97:1215-1216, 1953.
4. Des Saints, Sister Michel: Control of exposure to radiation, X-ray Technician 34:214-217, 1963.
5. Deutschberger, O.: Fluoroscopy in diagnostic roentgenology, Philadelphia, 1955, W. B. Saunders Co., chaps. 2, 7.
6. G. E. X-ray Corporation, Technical Service Department: Medical Radiographic technic, Springfield, Ill., 1944, Charles C Thomas, Publisher, chaps. VI, VII, XII, XV.
7. Greenfield, M. A.: Current status of radiation hazards, X-ray Technician 33:406-410, 1962.
8. Harmer, B., and Henderson, V.: Textbook of the principles and practice of nursing, New York, 1955, The Macmillan Co., chaps. 8, 25, 26, and pp. 601-604.
9. Hine, G. J., and Brownell, G. L.: Radiation dosimetry, New York, 1956, Academic Press, Inc.
10. Hull, E., and Perrodin, C.: Medical nursing, ed. 4, Philadelphia, 1952, F. A. Davis Co., chap. 49.
11. Jaffke, R. C.: Some sound advice in x-ray protection, X-ray Technician 24:34, 1952.

12. Kirsch, I. E.: Useful precautions in radiography from the genetic point of view, J.A.M.A. **164:**553-554, 1957.
13. Lachman, E.: Dangers of diagnostic radiation and protective measures, X-Ray Technician **25:**331, 1954.
14. Marvin, J. F.: Radiation protection for the technician in training, Minnesota Med. **39:**240-241, 1946.
15. McClain, M. E., and Gragg, S. H.: Scientific principles in nursing, ed. 5, St. Louis, 1966, The C. V. Mosby Co.
16. McNeill, C.: Roentgen technique, Springfield, Ill., 1947, Charles C Thomas, Publisher, part IV.
17. Merrill, V.: Atlas of roentgenographic positions, ed. 3, Vol. 1, St. Louis, 1967, The C. V. Mosby Co.
18. Meschan, I.: Roentgen signs in clinical diagnosis, Philadelphia, 1952, W. B. Saunders Co., pp. 24-29.
19. Moeller, D. W., and others: Radiation exposure in the United States, Public Health Rep. **68:**57-65, 1953.
20. Montag, M. L., and Swenson, R. P. S.: Fundamentals in nursing care, ed. 3, Philadelphia, 1959, W. B. Saunders Co., chaps. 16, 30, 31.
21. Naterman, H. L., and Robins, J. A.: Cutaneous test with Diodrast to predict allergic systemic reactions from Diodrast given intravenously, J.A.M.A. **119:**491-493, 1942.
22. Okel, E.: Opaque media, X-ray Technician **24:**337, 1953.
23. Ott, T. T.: Radiation protection in cerebroangiography, X-ray Technician **25:**46, 1953.
24. Pendergrass, E. P., Chamberlain, G. W., Godfrey, J. W., and Burdick, E. D.: A survey of deaths and unfavorable sequelae following administration of contrast media, Amer. J. Roentgen. **48:**741, 1942.
25. Perra, C. A.: May's manual of the diseases of the eye, ed. 20, Baltimore, 1949, The Williams & Wilkins Co., pp. 20-21.
26. Protection of x-ray personnel, Med. Tech. Bull. Suppl. U. S. Armed Forces M. J. **3:**68-69, 1952.
27. Rigler, L. G.: Outline of roentgen diagnosis, Atlas edition, Philadelphia, 1938, J. B. Lippincott Co., section 1.
28. Sante, L. R.: Manual of roentgenological technique, Ann Arbor, Mich., 1945, Edwards Bros., Inc., chaps. VI, VII, X, XIII.
29. Sherman, R. S.: Diagnostic radiology and radiation exposure, Health News **34:**16-19, 1957.
30. Singer, A. G., Jr.: Comparison of intradermal and ocular methods of testing for sensitivity of Diodrast, Amer. J. Roentgen. **59:**727, 1948.
31. Starch, C. B.: Fundamentals of clinical fluoroscopy, New York, 1951, Grune & Stratton, Inc., chap. 1.
32. The biological effects of atomic radiation, Washington, D. C., 1956, National Academy of Sciences, National Research Council.
33. The effects of atomic weapons, Los Alamos Scientific Laboratory. Prepared for and in Cooperation with the U. S. Dept. of Defense and the U. S. Atomic Energy Commission, Sept., 1950, Government Printing Office.
34. Walker, B. D.: Contrast media, X-ray Technician **30:**380-384, 1959.

Chapter 5

The technician and special patient care

BEDSIDE RADIOGRAPHY
Hospital ward procedure

There are some patients who are not always able to come to the x-ray department for radiography because of the nature of their illness or condition. However, the technician is confronted with similar problems associated with their special care, regardless of whether the x-ray picture is taken at the bedside or in the department.

Each condition will be discussed separately, but first some suggestions (basic hospital procedure) are given to help the technician function smoothly on the wards so that the patient is disrupted the least and the optimum quality of care is given.

1. The technician should always report to the nurse in *charge* on the ward, station, or floor. This may be the head nurse, her assistant, or another graduate nurse who is responsible for the patients. There are four reasons why the technician should do this. First, the charge nurse should always be kept informed of activity on her ward; second, she can correctly direct the technician to the patient's room and bed; third, she can enlist another nurse, aide, or orderly to help if it is necessary; and fourth, she can tell the technician anything specific that should or should not be done with the patient (Fig. 5-1).

2. The suggestions listed earlier about the technician's attitude and manner, proper explanation, providing privacy, comfort, and safety should be remembered.

3. Before the x-ray machine is wheeled in, the technician should go in, greet the patient with a smile, introduce herself, and explain what she is going to do. It is not only mystifying but also disturbing and unpleasant for a patient to see a huge piece of equipment being pushed into the room, not knowing what it is for.

4. If the patient is in a private room, the door should be closed. If he is in a double room or ward, the cubicle curtains should be drawn or screens placed in position to provide privacy.

5. The technician should remember the directions and warnings the charge nurse gave concerning the patient—that the bed should not be lowered, that he is hard of hearing, that he is blind, that he should not be turned to the left, or other similar instructions.

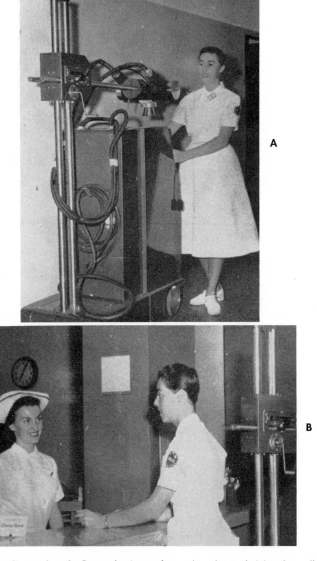

Fig. 5-1. Portable radiography. **A,** Remembering safety rules, the technician has all projecting parts of the machine out of the way, has good control of the machine, and walks on the right side of the corridor. **B,** The technician reports to the charge nurse before any bedside radiography. She will receive instructions on a patient's location, any precautions in positioning him, and any extra help if it is required.

6. Lifting and moving of the patient should be done safely and comfortably for him and the technician, and the aforementioned rules on body mechanics, patient comfort, and safety recalled.

7. After the x-ray picture has been taken and the patient is covered and comfortable, the technician should report back to the charge nurse to inform her that the film has been taken.

Problems of portable radiography

Limits of x-ray equipment. Portable or bedside x-ray equipment is generally available in 15 Ma., 30 Ma., 100 Ma., 200 Ma., and 300 Ma. capacities. The larger capacity units have autotransformer kilovoltages available up to 125 KVP. The units most commonly found in the average hospital are the 100 Ma. and 200 Ma. units. If a hospital is new and if thoughtful planning has been used, greater capacity mobile x-ray units may have been purchased. There also may be available, within the reach of every bed, the 220-volt circuits necessary to utilize these larger machines.

In the higher capacity equipment, milliamperage and kilovoltage can be varied to maintain very short exposure times. But in the average portable unit available in most hospitals, time becomes the most important variable, with the result that in every instance a longer exposure time is necessary for each film than would be necessary if conventional x-ray equipment were being used. This problem may be likened to fast photography with an inexpensive box camera as compared to the same photography with an expensive camera and an extremely fast lens. For example, in taking a film of a person diving, using the expensive, fast lens type of camera, one could stop the motion on the picture and have a photograph of a person suspended in midair in the process of the dive. With the inexpensive box camera and an inexpensive type lens, one would have a blur which would represent the person falling toward the water. This then is true also in x-ray films made with the low capacity equipment as compared to the high capacity equipment. The high capacity equipment allows a fast enough exposure time to stop motion, whereas the low capacity equipment will very often give a blurred radiograph, lacking in detail.

It is obvious then that the single, most important handicap in producing radiographs with portable equipment is the lack of capacity of the equipment. This becomes much less a handicap, however, when electrical circuits with a capacity of 220 volts are provided within reach of all hospital beds to permit the use of heavy mobile units. The wire size of the electrical leads to the 220 volt circuit should be 00 with a suitable ground. This type of power supply would permit the use of 100, 200, or 300 Ma. portable x-ray equipment. The technician would then have units at command which would permit extremely fast exposure times. Since the results of a radiograph often dictate the course of treatment of a patient, it would follow that better and more efficient patient care and treatment could be achieved if proper planning occurred during the construction of a hospital. In the event an x-ray technician is consulted during the building of a new hospital, information of this type made available to the architect may result in saving patients' lives by permitting better radiographs when the hospital is put into operation.

Precautions and hazards of the power supply. Inadequate electrical circuits can complicate patient care.

Capacity. Most of the older hospitals in the United States have been inadequately wired considering the enormous electrical load these wires are required to bear. The latter is due to the vast increase in the use of electrical apparatus in hospital care without a comparable increase in power supply to handle this apparatus. In many hospital rooms one will find the so-called octopus plugs. This type of multiple plug requires the electrical circuits to attempt to supply more power than is available within the circuit. When the requirements of a portable x-ray machine are added to the already overloaded circuit, there may be dangerous results. A fuse may be blown the minute the exposure switch is turned on in the x-ray circuit. If suction apparatus, oxygen tents, or other electrical equipment is being used on the same circuit, an immediate emergency will result insofar as the patient's treatment is concerned. It is well, therefore, for the x-ray department to obtain from the hospital engineering staff some idea of the power loads used in various areas of the hospital. Then if a portable x-ray film is required in this area, power supply for the x-ray machine might be provided by disconnecting electrical apparatus which *can* be interrupted without harm to the patient for the space of time necessary to do the radiograph.

Reliability. Another function of power supply is to ensure the reliability of an x-ray machine. If it is being used on an inadequate power supply, a lighter photographic effect may result even though it is being used at its capacity. For example, a portable chest film may be attempted with a 15 Ma. mobile x-ray unit at 75 KVP, at ¼ second at 15 Ma. This would result in an exposure of 4 Ma. seconds, approximately at 75 KVP. If the resulting radiograph were too light for diagnostic purposes, the technician might well go back to the patient's room and attempt another radiograph using 80 KVP at 15 Ma. at ½ second. However, even with *increased* factors, with an inadequate power supply the resultant radiograph might well be lighter than the radiograph made with the *lesser* factors. Cutting the milliamperage and increasing the exposure time is the proper procedure when an overloaded line is indicated. Quite often if an overloaded line is a complicating factor, a radiograph made at ½ second at 8 Ma. at 75 KVP or 4 Ma. seconds at 75 KVP will have a much greater density than a radiograph made at 15 Ma. at ¼ second at 75 KVP, which is also 4 Ma. seconds at 75 KVP. The reason for this phenomenon is that when the portable equipment is used at its rated capacities it may be demanding more power supply than is available in the circuit. Electrical power supply will try to meet demands up to its capacity. When it goes beyond its capacity, a law similar to the law of diminishing returns becomes effective. This is a complicating factor that the x-ray technician cannot do much about except to be aware of and know how to compromise with it.

RADIOGRAPHY OF PATIENTS WHO REQUIRE SPECIAL CARE
Care of the surgical patient

General considerations. The patient who has had surgery is often approached with a little fear, hesitancy, and reluctance by the technician until he has had repeated experience in handling and lifting him and in caring for him with all tubes, drainage bottles, intravenous feedings, and dressings necessary for his care.

Parenteral fluids. These are fluids that are given to a patient through any route other than by mouth. Naturally, a patient who has had abdominal surgery or gastrointestinal surgery will not be able to eat for a certain time following the operation, allowing his wound, inside and out, to heal. Neither can the unconscious person eat. In these instances and others, the patient is nourished by giving him fluids by another route, either directly into his vein, intravenous feeding (I.V.), or into his subcutaneous tissues (Subq.). Parenteral fluids are

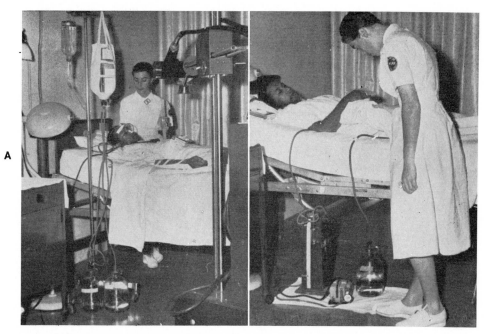

A   **B**

Fig. 5-2. The surgical patient. **A,** The technician must determine where the portable machine can be placed, considering the patient's immobilized arm where he is receiving an intravenous feeding and his nasal tube and suction apparatus. She must remember to roll him *toward* his tubing and not to jar any of the bottles with the x-ray machine. **B,** The technician is wise in assessing the situation of the surgical patient. Care must be taken in positioning so that the tubings in either the chest suction or urinary retention catheter systems are not pulled out or become separated.

often given to patients who *can* swallow and eat but who need supplementary nourishment to prepare them for surgery or build them up physically (Fig. 5-2, *A*). Sometimes certain medicines are administered this way.

Blood, plasma, distilled water with sugar or glucose added to make a 5 or 10% solution, and distilled water with salt added to make a 0.9% solution are most often used. Patients frequently receive 2 to 3 quarts of solution a day until their condition is improved. The solution drips into the patient's vein through a needle at a rate of about 45 drops a minute from a bottle hung upside down on a standard. The vein most often used is the one at the inner side of the elbow, although if a patient has received many intravenous feedings, his vein wall may become thickened and difficult to enter with a needle. Therefore, a vein in his wrist or hand may be used. In babies, a scalp vein is most often used. For subcutaneous fluids the most frequent sites for injection are the front of the thighs. Patients receiving parenteral fluids sometimes have the arm taped to a padded board to remind them not to bend the arm, although they can turn in bed, sit and get up, and are generally not restricted at all in their movement except that they cannot bend at the needle site.

If the patient is brought to the x-ray department, care must be taken when he is lifted to the x-ray table so that his intravenous bottle is moved with him and hung close by. The technician should guide his arm to offer more protection so that the needle will not be dislodged from the vein. If the technician goes to the station for a portable x-ray film, care must be taken to avoid hitting the intravenous bottle on the standard with the x-ray machine. In positioning, the patient must be rolled toward his tubing and bottle, rather than away from it, otherwise, there will not be enough slack tubing, and the strain on it may dislodge the needle.

The rate of flow of the parenteral fluid is never to be adjusted by the technician. Neither should the needle be withdrawn. If, however, the patient is in the department for any length of time, the technician *is* responsible for checking two things. First, the fluid should still be dripping at an even rate. If it is not, the technician should call the station charge nurse who will probably ask the technician to clamp the tube, *not* pull out the needle. Second, the arm should occasionally be checked at the site of the needle. It should appear no different from usual. However, if the needle has been dislodged from the patient's vein during his journey to or his stay in the department, the tissue at the needle site will be white, puffy, and swollen. This means the fluid is seeping into the tissue around the vein and is called infiltration. The station charge nurse should be informed and will probably ask the technician to clamp off the fluid. These two observations can easily be made when a technician takes a portable film also, and anything adverse can be reported to the station charge nurse.

If at any time a needle is pulled completely out of a patient's vein, the technician should clamp off the tubing immediately so that no fluid flows out and is wasted. Pressure with a gauze square or tissue should be exerted for a minute or two at the site where the needle came out so the patient will not become black and blue from the blood oozing into the tissue. Prompt reporting to the charge nurse is essential. Then when the patient returns to the ward, the bottle of fluid must be sent with him, since accurate records are kept on the amount and kind of fluid the patient receives.

Gastric and intestinal suction. Frequently a surgical patient has a long tube inserted through his nose to his stomach or small bowel. The tube is attached to a suction apparatus, which draws out the contents of the stomach or intestines and collects this material in a trap bottle. When used before surgery, the suction's purpose may be to empty out the stomach, making it easier to operate. It is often used to remove trapped waste and gas in patient's bowel when, due to some disturbance, the passage in the bowel is blocked. The latter is called decompression. When such suction is used postoperatively, the purpose is to empty out the normal continuous secretions of the stomach or bowel, to promote healing, and to decrease nausea and gas formation (Fig. 5-2, *A*).

Some hospitals have wall suction and the patient's nasal tube is attached directly to the wall outlet. However, most hospitals still use the conventional suction method involving negative pressure and three bottles (Fig. 5-3). Bottle 1 is filled with water and hung upside down. As water gradually flows from it to Bottle 2 by gravity, a vacuum is created in the upper part of Bottle 1. This vacuum extends all the way through the patient's tube to his stomach or intestine, drawing out the contents and trapping them in Bottle 3. If a patient

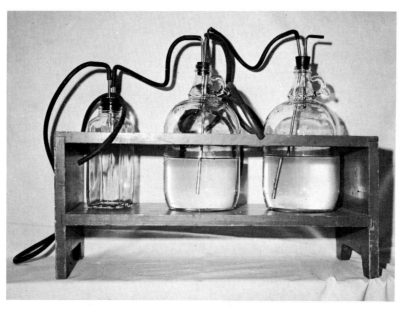

Fig. 5-3. Three-bottle intestinal suction.

comes to the x-ray department with all three bottles, care must be taken, as with the intravenous bottles, to move them with the patient and to keep the tube in Bottle 2 under water always. If it is not, the vacuum is broken and the system will have to be restarted. Most often the patient does not need constant suction and the short time he is in the department without nasal suction is not harmful. Therefore, before he goes to the x-ray department, the station nurse generally clamps his tube near his nose, thus keeping air out of his stomach, clamps the two tubes that close off the suction system, and disconnects the system.

When a portable x-ray film is taken, the technician must be careful not to hit any bottles with the x-ray machine and should ask the patient to roll over *toward* his tubing to prevent strain on it and irritation to the patient's nose. If all the water has flowed into Bottle 1, the technician should report it to the charge nurse, who will see that Bottles 1 and 2 are rotated and the system restarted.

Chest suction. There are occasions, following chest surgery, that tubes are placed in the patient's chest cavity and attached to suction to withdraw fluid or air from the space and help the lungs reexpand. Suction in this instance is usually electrical, because it must be a little stronger than mere mechanical suction, as in the aforementioned method. It is of utmost importance not to open the suction system by rolling the patient on to the glass section of tubing and breaking it or by pulling out a chest catheter. It is of equal importance not to interrupt the suction system by stepping on the tubing on the floor or rolling the machine over it. If the system is opened, air can easily enter the patient's chest and undo the good the suction has previously done, or it can retard his progress considerably. If a break in the system occurs, the technician must quickly clamp the patient's tube or tubes close to his body with a forceps or the fingers and call for immediate assistance. Almost always the charge nurse will assign someone to help the technician with the handling of these patients during the x-ray examination to assure him the safest and best care (Fig. 5-2, *B*).

T *Tubes.* Following gallbladder surgery, a surgeon often leaves a tube in the form of a T in the patient's biliary tract to promote drainage. The fluid is allowed merely to drip out, and the tube is not generally connected to any suction. The bottle to which the tubing is connected may be at the floor level, tied at bed level, or placed on the patient's bedside stand. The symptoms which the patient has when the biliary drainage ends at any of these levels give the doctors clues concerning his postsurgical progress. Care must be taken here, too, in positioning the patient so that he be rolled *toward* his slack tubing and bottle and so that the technician not break the bottle with the x-ray machine. This tube, like a nasal tube or a needle for parenteral fluids, cannot merely be reinserted on the station if it is pulled out accidentally. The patient must be taken to the operating room and the tube must be reinserted under general anesthetic, involving much more risk, time, and expense.

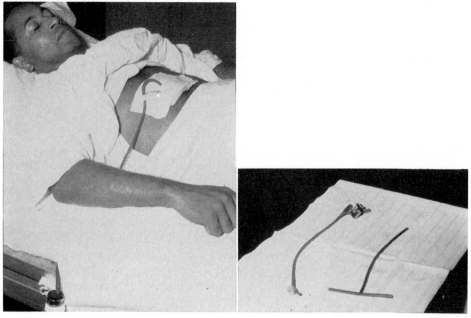

Fig. 5-4   **Fig. 5-5**

Fig. 5-4. The patient with a biliary T tube. The tube is pinned with adhesive to the dressing, decreasing tension on it, to reduce chances of its pulling out. If the pin will interfere with the x-ray, the technician must receive permission to remove it. The patient's tube drains into the bottle tied at mattress level.

Fig. 5-5. A urinary retention catheter and a T tube. After the catheter is inserted, water is injected through a separate small tube within the catheter to inflate the balloon, thus keeping the catheter in the bladder. A clamp is placed on this part keeping the water in and the balloon inflated. The crossbar of the T is placed in the hepatic duct and common bile duct, allowing bile to drain from the liver out the length of the tube to the patient's bottle.

Occasionally after a T tube has been inserted, it is held in place by a safety pin which is attached to adhesive around the tube and then pinned to adhesive on the patient's abdomen. If the pin will interfere with the area to be x-rayed, it can be removed only with consent of the surgeon or the radiologist, and it is removed by them, not by the technician (Figs. 5-4 and 5-5).

Rectal tubes. Rectal tubes, similar to ones used for enemas, are inserted to promote the expulsion of gas (flatus). Surgical patients often need rectal tubes since, due to tissue trauma during surgery, the normal peristaltic waves of the intestines are temporarily absent or slowed and gas collects causing distension. A gauze square is usually wrapped around the open end of the tube or else it is placed into a small cardboard container to hold any small amount of fecal matter that is passed. Usually the tube does not come out very easily, but if it does, it can be reinserted without difficulty by a nurse. However, the technician should still take precautions not to dislodge it, and after the x-ray examination is completed she should make sure that the tube is in the container or wrapper with the gauze square.

Urinary retention catheters. When a person is unable to void voluntarily for any of several reasons, a catheter is inserted through the urethra to the bladder so that continuous drainage of the urine can take place. If the patient had bladder surgery, a catheter may be inserted to keep the bladder walls collapsed and allow healing. A patient with any abdominal or pelvic operation may have a catheter inserted, since the muscles that control voiding are relaxed or may need to heal (Figs. 5-2, *B* and 5-5).

Precautions need to be taken when positioning or transporting patients with urinary catheters. These precautions are similar to those observed with patients who have nasal catheters and chest catheters, remembering that it is important to turn a patient toward his catheter and tubing to prevent its separating from the drainage bottle, thus causing a break in a sterile system. The urinary tract, unlike the gastrointestinal tract, is sterile, and if bacteria are allowed to enter, bladder or urinary tract infection could result. Another reason for careful turning is that undue tension of the catheter causes pain in the urethra. The tube is held in place by the inflation of a small balloon about ¾ inch in diameter, and it is this balloon being pulled down from the bladder into the urethra that causes pain.

If an x-ray picture of the pelvic area is ordered, the technician must be sure the clamp which is keeping the water in the balloon is not interfering with the x-ray picture. If the clamp, which is opaque, is lying over a part of the exposed area, it will interfere with a part of the film that is especially important. Care should be taken, too, that for comfort reasons, the patient is not lying on the clamp.

The technician must never disconnect the patient's catheter. If a catheter is to be disconnected, it is done by a nurse who knows the sterile technique that must be used and is aware of all the factors involved. If a patient's catheter is disconnected from the tubing by mistake, the technician should then clamp the patient's catheter so that urine does not continue to drip out, and she should immediately notify the charge nurse of the patient's station. The bottle of urine to which the tubing was connected must be returned to the station with the patient, since accurate urine output records are kept and play a part in determining the parenteral fluids ordered. If the catheter comes out completely, the technician should immediately call the station and inform the charge nurse, since upon the patient's return to the ward, a new sterile catheter will have to be reinserted.

Surgical dressings. The gauze, bandage, and pads that cover a patient's surgical wound are called dressings. Since they are of limited opacity they are generally not removed to take a film unless specifically ordered by the surgeon or the radiologist.

An exception is when a barium enema must be given to a patient through his colostomy. Colostomy patients have had surgery on the rectum and lower bowel and, either temporarily or permanently, have had the remaining end of the intestine transplanted to the outside of the abdomen. Through this small red piece of protruding bowel they expel their feces into clean dressings and pads. After several months a patient can learn, with diet and daily enemas, to control his bowel movements and have them regularly once a day, thus eliminating the need for dressings. When a barium enema is ordered for a patient with a colostomy, the technician can remove the dressings. It is wise to use clean rubber gloves or a clean forceps, not so much to prevent contamination of the wound, since, being a part of the gastrointestinal tract or bowel, it is not sterile, but rather to keep the technician's hands clean. The technique used for giving the barium enema will be described in a later section.

After certain types of surgery where a drainage from a wound may excoriate or irritate the surrounding skin, zinc or iodoform paste often is applied around the wound by the doctor or nurse before the dressings are applied. Most commonly this is done for a patient with a colostomy, an ileostomy, or with the aforementioned biliary surgery where a T tube is left in place. If an abdominal x-ray examination is ordered for these patients and the radiologist orders the dressings removed, then the technician must make sure that the zinc paste or iodoform gauze is also removed since it is opaque and will interfere with the x-ray picture. The paste can be removed most effectively by pouring a small amount of mineral oil into a medicine glass or basin and wiping off the zinc paste with cotton balls dipped into the mineral oil. The technician can do this for the patient who has the colostomy, since sterile technique need not be used. After the film is taken, for this type of patient, a clean gauze square or pad should be placed over the wound until the surgeon, radiologist, or nurse can dress it.

The radiologist will remove the dressings on a patient with a T tube, clean off the area, and temporarily redress it, since the area involved here is a sterile one and precautions need to be taken so as not to infect the wound.

If a patient's surgical dressings, whether they cover his head, abdomen, chest, or any other part of the body, appear wet, the technician must avoid touching them. The purpose of surgical dressings is to prevent bacteria from entering the patient's incision or wound, and they are effective only so long as they are dry. Bacteria travel quickly along a wet area; if the dressings are wet at all, bacteria from the outer part of the dressings can enter the wound. The technician should not only avoid touching the wet dressings but should also reinforce them by placing a sterile pad over the bandages (Fig. 5-6). The technique that must be used to do this is described in the section on sterile technique and surgical asepsis.

The purpose of some dressings is not surgical but rather medical. In certain skin conditions, dressings are soaked with mercurial solutions to promote healing. Since they are opaque and will impair visualization, they should be removed, permission having been obtained from the attending physician. The technician

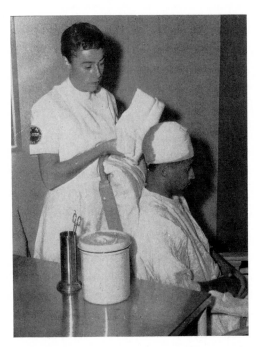

Fig. 5-6. Reinforcing a patient's head dressing. The technician has removed a sterile pad from a container and is placing it over a wet dressing. She can then tape it down, reinforcing it and keeping contamination at a minimum until the dressing can be changed completely at the patient's ward.

can remove them, but the nursing department is responsible for reapplication of the medical dressings.

In the x-ray department with which the author is associated, use is made of a red card pinned to the patient's gown after the x-ray examination stating whether dressings have been removed. It is possible that the patient's wound may remain undressed or improperly dressed for a short time unless the station nurses are aware of his situation. By informing, at a glance, with the eye-catching card, the dressings can be reapplied promptly when the patient returns.

Specific considerations. The aforementioned suggestions should always be remembered when caring for *any* surgical patient. However, further care must be taken with surgical patients who have had any of the following types of surgery:

Craniotomy. The patient with a craniotomy has had brain surgery which has necessitated opening his skull. He usually is kept in a sitting position, his bed is rarely lowered, and he may not lie down without the specific permission of his doctor. The patient may also have some weakness or paralysis, and the technician should be aware of its extent in order that the patient may be moved more safely and intelligently.

Leg amputation. The patient who has had a leg amputation must be rolled toward the side of the amputation, rather than away from it, to aid him in balancing and the control of his body. The bed should not be jarred with the x-ray machine and the stump must not be moved unnecessarily because of the intense pain it causes.

Eye surgery. In taking x-ray films of a patient who has had eye surgery, the technician should know which eye is involved. It is safe to work only from the opposite side of the bed. When a patient has had right eye surgery, the medical team members must work from the left side of the bed—in bathing him, examining him, taking films, and any other procedure. When the patient has a detached retina, the technician must have adequate help in positioning the patient so that he is disturbed as little as possible.

Tracheotomy. On occasion, a technician may take an x-ray film of a patient with either a temporary or a permanent interruption of his windpipe or trachea. This necessitates the patient's breathing or coughing through a small metal tube, called a tracheotomy tube, which has been surgically inserted through a hole in the neck into the trachea.

The tracheotomized patient can usually talk by placing a finger over the tube's opening, allowing outbreathed air to bypass it, pass through the larynx or voice box and thus emit sound. For these patients the interruption is a temporary one, perhaps to facilitate breathing in extensive oral or neck surgery or in tracheal obstruction. The tube is later removed and the hole in the neck is allowed to heal.

Laryngectomy. The laryngectomized patient, however, is one who has had his larynx removed. He is not able to talk, even were he to put a finger over the opening. His only means of communication is to write with pad and pencil. The laryngectomy tube is his only airway for breathing and it is a matter of life or death to keep it open. Any signs of choking or difficult breathing must be reported immediately to the charge nurse.

Care of the psychiatric patient

Department radiography. A psychiatric patient's actions and behavior may deviate from those of his fellow men because he is suffering from a mental disease, a disorder of the personality. There are many different kinds of mental disease, some mild and some serious. Symptoms are different and develop gradually. Mental disease needs early diagnosis and medical treatment just like any other disease.

It is important that the technician be no more fearful of a psychiatric patient than of a patient with lung, bone, or gastric disease. Sometimes the technician may be very aware that the patient is depressed or confused, that he is restless and agitated, imagining voices or sounds or visions, or that his conversation is garbled, but frequently this kind of patient shows no evidence of his illness.

Generally the psychiatric patient is brought to the x-ray department by a nurse or orderly. The films are usually skull films. He is never left alone or untended. The nurse or orderly always stays with him.

Bedside radiography. If the patient is severely disturbed, a portable film is taken on the ward. A nurse meets the technician at the locked door of the station and not only provides help but also informs her of any rules that must be observed in that particular area for the patient's own safety and protection. The care of this type of patient is like the care of emotionally disturbed patients which was described in Chapter 3. Portable radiography of the emotionally disturbed patient presents a great challenge. There are many approaches to the making of a radiograph on this type of patient. Anesthesia sometimes is used, quite often sedation is used, and in some instances restraints have been used. Any of these approaches is often contraindicated. Attending physicians will be reluctant to use anesthesia as a method of quieting a patient because of the complications that exist and the risks involved any time a patient undergoes general anesthesia. If the physician in charge of the patient should decide that the x-ray film is of sufficient importance to justify general anesthesia and there is no other method by which the patient may be quieted for a sufficient length of time to obtain films, he may authorize this type of procedure.

Despite the fact that the patient is under general anesthesia it is not wise to move him to the main department and back to his room. Bedside radiography is the preferred method for completing the examination. In cases of this nature the physician in charge and the anesthesiologist should be aware of the technical problems involved in making the requested radiograph. They in turn can govern their decision as to what is required in the line of cooperation from the patient and can evaluate whether the patient can possibly give this kind of cooperation without general anesthesia. The use of anesthesia as an immobilizing device is rarely used in radiography and then only if all other possibilities of obtaining the necessary films have been exhausted.

The use of sedation with the emotionally disturbed patient is a common approach to this problem but unfortunately is not too satisfactory, since dosages in sufficient amounts to control the patient are often prohibitive from the standpoint of medical treatment.

The use of restraints will permit obtaining the requested radiograph, but all too often this type of maneuver causes more excitement on the part of the patient. And even the restrained patient will be able to cause sufficient motion on the radiograph made with a portable x-ray unit to make such a radiograph unsatisfactory.

The best approach to this problem and the one that should always be the first used is a combination of technician ingenuity, cooperation with the nursing staff, and careful preparation before the procedure is attempted. An example of technician ingenuity in such a hospital is cited. A very disturbed female patient confined to her room and under partial restraint required a chest film.

The patient was intelligent and well educated. Several female x-ray technicians attempted to obtain the required x-ray. In each instance they made the proper approach to the problem by obtaining the assistance of the charge nurse, but immediately upon bringing the mobile equipment into the room the patient became violently disturbed, offered no cooperation, and would not permit the chest film to be made. Finally, the technician questioned the advisability of using the services of the male orderly rather than the nurses. The equipment was taken to the patient's room and she watched preparation for the examination with interest and with no show of emotion. When she was requested to cooperate during the film exposure, the film was made with no difficulty. A little investigation disclosed that this patient had an antipathy toward women, as a part of her illness, but did not resent the male staff. The orderly had been able to obtain cooperation from her previously, as had a male nurse and her physician. Any male technician could have made this radiograph with little trouble. This emphasizes the importance for the technician to discuss with the nurse or doctor the background of each emotionally disturbed patient with the idea of obtaining cooperation from the patient if at all possible.

Complete preparation before entering the patient's room is vital. The patient's chart which is available on the station will indicate his height and weight. The technician should then set up the mobile equipment, using this information to determine proper technical factors. After having obtained as much background information as possible about the patient, she should enter the room, introduce herself and briefly explain what is to be done. The equipment must be brought into the room with as little disturbance as possible and every attempt to reason with the patient should be made. Often they are apprehensive, confusing the x-ray machine with shock treatment. The nurse who has had the patient under her care and in whom the patient has confidence should be aware of what is expected and should explain this to the patient to prepare him. The technician must control his or her emotions and refrain from expressing impatience regardless of the difficulty of making the radiograph. Several attempts are often necessary on a patient of this sort.

Care of the paralyzed or physically handicapped patient

There are some illnesses that leave patients paralyzed—sometimes partially and sometimes almost completely. The paraplegic patient is one whose legs or lower body is paralyzed. The hemiplegic patient is paralyzed on a whole side of his body, and a quadriplegic is one who is paralyzed from the neck down. A cerebral accident or stroke, poliomyelitis, or a spinal injury are some of the conditions that can result in paralysis, since they attack or involve the central nervous system.

When these patients are brought to the x-ray department or when the technician goes to the ward with a portable x-ray machine, the extent to which the patient is assisted or the number of people needed to move him should be gauged

according to his disability. The paralyzed limb must be lifted gently and carefully, it should never be allowed to drag or get caught between the litter and the
x-ray table, and it should be kept in proper alignment. In poliomyelitis where
there is not only paralysis but also painful muscle spasm, even greater care and
gentleness in handling the limb should be considered.

Some hospitals now have special wards or stations where the medical team
is devoted to rehabilitation of a patient who is paralyzed. With time and patience, skill and determination, the patient and the team, in many instances, can
work together to help him back to independency. He must be guided slowly
and as new muscle groups are gradually trained to do a certain skill, he should
be allowed to practice this new skill even though it could be done in a much
shorter time by the nurse or team member. It is the technician's responsibility
then, as part of the medical team, to follow the charge nurse's suggestions when
she reports to her on the wards or the suggestions of the relative or nurse who
brings the patient to the department. If the patient has recently learned to lift
his leg, turn his arm, or raise his hand, he must be allowed to do it himself even
though it will take longer. The patient does not want sympathy or dependency.
It is up to the technician not to mistake helpfulness with interference in the plan
for recovery and rehabilitation. The best results are obtained with these patients
by working *with* them, not *on* them.

Care of the patient with a communicable disease

General considerations. The practice of general hygiene by the technician
has already been mentioned as exceedingly important in preventing the spread
of disease. Careful handwashing between care of patients, turning one's head to
cough or sneeze into a handkerchief, providing clean sheets and pillowcases for
every patient, and wearing clean uniforms are all important and are only some
of the aforementioned principles of general hygiene which, when practiced, help
to provide a safe environment for the patient.

However, while these principles should apply to all patients, extra precautions need to be taken in caring for patients with communicable diseases. The
utilization of all these principles and precautions to keep anything contaminated
by the patient from contact with anyone or anything else is called medical asepsis.

Communicable diseases are caused by bacteria or viruses. Some of the more
common communicable diseases with which the technician may have experience
in the hospital are pneumonia, poliomyelitis, meningitis, and tuberculosis. Children with the communicable diseases common to childhood—measles, mumps,
scarlet fever, whooping cough, and others—are sometimes admitted to hospitals,
although in recent years these patients are not hospitalized unless there are
complications.

An organism's ability to invade the body and cause infection depends on the
virulence or power of the organism and the person's resistance. This resistance
or lack of susceptibility to a disease is called immunity. It can be *natural* im-

munity where the person is born with resistance to a certain disease. Or it can be *acquired* immunity—acquired in an *active* way by having the disease once, by being repeatedly exposed to it, or by injecting small amounts of the weakened organism (vaccination). Active immunity leaves the person with antibodies to protect him from the same disease again. Acquired immunity can also be *passive*. When *another* person's antibodies are introduced into the blood, resistance to that particular disease is acquired. This is not to be confused with vaccination, where the weakened disease organism itself is introduced into the patient and the patient himself produces the antibodies.

Disease organisms can enter the body through three main channels: the respiratory tract, the gastrointestinal tract, and the skin. The spread can be by *direct* contact, from the infected person directly to another person. Sneezing or coughing (droplet infections) are examples of spread by direct contact.

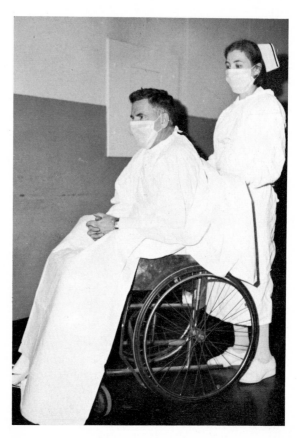

Fig. 5-7. Patient with a communicable disease. When this patient is brought to the x-ray department for radiography, every precaution is taken to keep the contamination confined to his person. The wheel chair is protected with a sheet, and the technician is pushing it with her hands under the sheet. If waiting is necessary, the patient should be kept apart from other patients.

Spread can also be by *indirect* contact, from the infected person to another person with something else as the "middleman." The five most frequent "middlemen" are called the Five F's: fingers, flies, feces, food, and fomites, the latter being inanimate objects like doorknobs, x-ray tables, drinking cups, and soiled toys or bed linen.

Patients who have a communicable disease should be isolated from other patients—either in a single room or in a ward with other patients having the same disease. Everything in the unit or room is considered contaminated. Regardless of where the patient is cared for, the room or unit is considered a contaminated area, and all techniques are carried out with one purpose in mind, that of preventing the infectious organism from being carried out of the area.

Departmental radiography. Taking x-ray pictures of these patients presents unusual problems to the technician. If the patient is brought to the x-ray department, protection of other patients and of the technicians must be considered (Fig. 5-7).

1. The charge nurse should never be called to send the patient to the department until the technician is ready. When the patient arrives, his x-ray picture should be taken immediately. If, due to some unfortunate emergency, he must wait a few minutes, he should wait in an area away from the other patients.

2. If the disease is spread through the air (droplet infection), the patient can wear a mask and no one else will need to do so. Or, if a mask is not worn by the patient, masks must be worn by the nurse or aide transporting him as well as by all other people in the x-ray department with whom the patient comes in contact.

3. The nurse or aide who brings the patient will wear a gown if she must touch the patient at all—assist him to the table, position him, etc. After she has once come in contact with the patient, she is "contaminated," and anything she touches will also be contaminated.

4. The technician must wear a gown if she has to assist the patient or position him in any way; otherwise just the mask is sufficient.

5. The patient will be brought to the department in a wheel chair or on a litter which is first covered by a clean sheet. The "patient" side of the sheet is contaminated, but the under side touching the chair or litter is not. Care must be taken so that the contaminated side does not touch the x-ray table. If the sheet becomes wet, it is entirely contaminated.

6. To protect the table, a clean sheet can be placed on it, upon which the patient can lie.

7. If the technician has contaminated herself in any way, she must not touch the x-ray machine until she has washed her hands thoroughly for 2 minutes. Therefore, it is wise to have two technicians on hand for patients with a communicable disease—one to stay "clean" and the other to help the patient and be "contaminated."

8. After the x-ray picture has been taken, the contaminated linen will need

special care. (a) It can be returned with the patient to his room to be disposed of in his contaminated area. (b) Or a "clean" technician will bring a *striped* bag, or one plainly marked "contaminated" into which the "contaminated" technician drops her mask, her gown, and the sheet that was on the table. This is different from the disposal of a gown, mask, and sheet used for infants who do not have a communicable disease. The materials used in their care may be discarded with the regular linen. The gown and mask worn in the latter instance is to protect the *baby* from any disease, whereas in caring for patients with communicable disease, the gown and mask are worn to protect the *personnel* and other patients from a contagious disease.

9. If during the taking of the film the x-ray table, stool, and any equipment becomes contaminated, they must be thoroughly scrubbed with a disinfectant or soap and water.

10. The "contaminated" technician and anyone who came into contact with the patient or his linen must wash her hands and arms thoroughly under running water, rinsing and soaping frequently for 2 minutes. If the sink has hand faucets, she must turn them on with a paper towel so that they do not become contaminated, and then discard the towel in the wastebasket.

Bedside radiography. When a portable x-ray machine must be taken to a patient in isolation, two technicians or one technician and one nurse must be assigned. One plans to become "contaminated" and wears a gown and mask. The other remains "clean" but wears a mask if she goes into the patient's room. A suggested procedure is described as follows:

1. After reporting to the charge nurse, a clean pillowcase and a large sheet should be obtained from the station linen room.

2. From the supply of clean gowns on the table outside the patient's room, the technician who will become contaminated takes one and puts it on, carefully covering her uniform (Fig. 5-8). This method of using a gown only once and then disposing of it is preferred. An alternate method of hanging a gown after use and then reusing it is rarely used, because it offers too great an opportunity for spread of infection.

3. Both technicians put on a mask, looping the upper ties over the ears, typing them under the chin, and bringing the lower ties behind the neck, making a bow. There is much controversy about the effectiveness of masks. Some hospital staffs agree that they are of little value, since bacteria can freely pass through after the mask becomes moist from breathing. Therefore, the technician must abide by the rules of the hospital in which she works. In any event, to wear a mask incorrectly is a greater hazard than not to wear one at all. Masks should not be worn for long periods of time, and, after use, must be removed, not left to dangle around the neck.

4. Before entering with the machine, one of the technicians goes into the patient's room, without touching anything, and explains to the patient what is to be done. The machine then can be wheeled in.

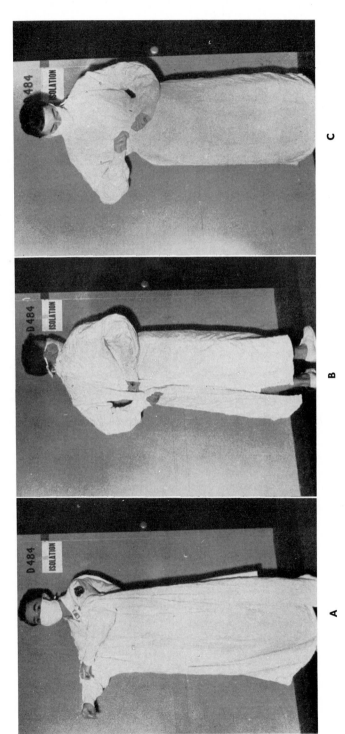

A   B   C

Fig. 5-8. Gowning for care of a patient with a communicable disease. **A,** The gown is put on, keeping it above floor level. **B,** The technician pulls it around in back, careful to cover all parts of her uniform. **C,** The gown is tied securely in front.

5. The "contaminated" technician positions the patient, at this point contaminating herself, and moves any furniture so the "clean" technician can plug in the machine. After the "contaminated" technician has once touched the patient or anything in his room or unit, she must not touch the machine or the "clean" technician (Fig. 5-9, *A*).

6. The "clean" technician lays the clean sheet over the patient's bed and rolls

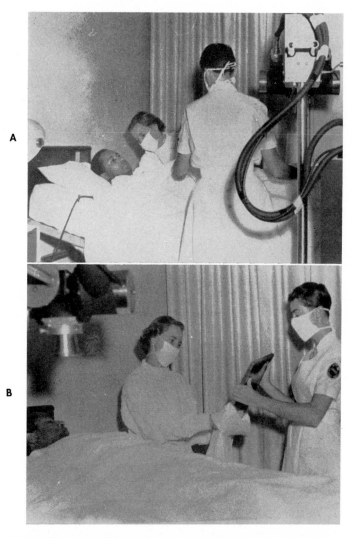

Fig. 5-9. Bedside radiography of the isolated patient. **A,** Both technicians wear masks. The "contaminated" technician has the gown on and is positioning the patient, while the "clean" technician places a clean sheet over the bed to protect the machine. **B,** After the procedure is completed, the "contaminated" technician holds the pillowcase in such a way that the "clean" technician can reach down into it and remove the cassette without contaminating it or herself.

the machine up to the bed, thus protecting the machine from contamination (Fig. 5-9, *A*).

7. She drops the cassette into the clean pillowcase, folds the case over, and hands it to the "contaminated" technician, who places it in position.

8. The "clean" technician makes the exposure, after which the "contaminated" technician withdraws the covered cassette from the patient, and holds the pillowcase wide open so the "clean" technician can reach in and draw out the cassette. (Fig. 5-9, *B*).

9. The "contaminated" technician makes the patient comfortable, removes the sheet from the patient's bed and drops it into the linen bag or hamper *in* the patient's room.

10. Before she leaves the room, she removes her gown. She unties the strings at the waist and loosens the gown, pulls one of her sleeves inside out so that the clean side of the gown is outermost, unties the string at the neck. She removes the gown, completely holding it away from her, and drops it in the striped or contaminated bag or hamper in the patient's room (Fig. 5-10).

11. With her mask still on, she goes out of the room to a sink in the hall marked "isolation" and there washes her hands and arms for 2 minutes under running water, soaping and rinsing frequently. Since the faucets are already con-

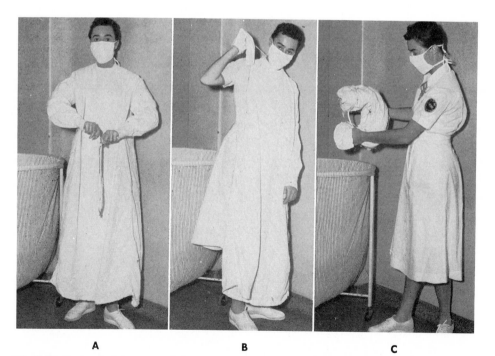

| A | B | C |

Fig. 5-10. Removal of the gown. **A**, The gown is untied in front. **B**, Pulling the arm of the gown inside out, the technician uses the "clean" inner side to reach around and untie the neck tapes. **C**, The technician removes the gown, holding it away from her, and discards it in the hamper in the patient's room.

taminated, she should use a paper towel to turn them off. This is different from the procedure in the x-ray department where the sink is not contaminated.

12. After she has "scrubbed," she removes her mask and drops it into a small bag for masks marked "contaminated" at the door of the patient's room. She must make sure the mask strings are also inside the bag.

13. After the "clean" technician has taken the cassette she can leave it outside the patient's room on the table, but not on the floor, which is grossly contaminated. A cleaning rag or gauze can be obtained from the charge nurse and soaked with a disinfectant. With this, she reenters the patient's unit and grasps the cord of the x-ray machine, the only part of the machine which has become contaminated since it was on the floor. With the disinfectant soaked cloth, she scrubs it, being careful not to contaminate herself on the furniture in the patient's room or to contaminate the cord by letting it drop on the floor again after it has been cleaned. She can then discard this cloth in the linen bag in the patient's room.

14. After removing the machine from the room, she can remove her mask and return to the main department, after first reporting back to the charge nurse.

This method of isolation technique can be adapted to various situations, and the procedure carried out safely with a few deviations *if* the technician has a good understanding of medical asepsis—what is contaminated and what is not. It is no great catastrophe if something does become contaminated if the technician is aware that it *is* contaminated and takes precautions to prevent further spread of infection. For instance, if the machine did become contaminated during the procedure, mere scrubbing with a disinfectant would remedy the situation.

Often patients isolated physically from others due to a communicable disease are also isolated psychologically and are lonesome, anxious people. A pleasant voice and manner go a long way. The technician should avoid being reluctant in handling the patient as if he were an "untouchable." Hands always can be washed after contact with him. Machines and cassettes can always be scrubbed, too. Technique and medical asepsis should not be emphasized so much that the technician forgets the patient.

Standard isolation technique is an attempt to prevent the spreading of disease by isolating the patient who has this disease. There is, however, the problem of reverse isolation. In this instance, the patient does not have a communicable disease, but due to a variety of reasons he may be very susceptible to acquiring disease. For example, a patient in shock, a patient who is very ill with cancer, or a patient who is postoperative from major surgery will have a lowered resistance to any disease. If one was to do portable radiography on such a patient, it would be necessary for any technicians or nurses concerned with the examination to follow isolation techniques as far as they personally are concerned, and in this instance, it is necessary to prevent the spread of any disease germs they may be carrying to the patient who, at the time, has a very low resistance to infection. The same criteria must be applied in handling newborn patients when they require radiographic examinations.

REFERENCES

Care of the surgical patient

1. Bird, B.: Psychological aspects of preoperative-postoperative care, Amer. J. Nur. **55:** 685-687, 1955.
2. Brown, A. F.: Medical nursing, ed. 3, Philadelphia, 1957, W. B. Saunders Co., pp. 474-484.
3. Cantor, M. O.: Intestinal intubation, Springfield, Ill., 1949, Charles C Thomas, Publisher.
4. Clotworthy, H. W., Jr., and Stewart, M. M.: Intravenous therapy for infants and children, Amer. J. Nurs. **57:**630, 1957.
5. Conley, J. J.: Tracheotomy, Amer. J. Nurs. **52:**1078-1081, 1952.
6. Davis, L.: Christopher's textbook of surgery, Philadelphia, 1956, W. B. Saunders Co., chaps. 5, 12, 13.
7. Eliason, E., Ferguson, L. K., and Sholtis: Surgical nursing, ed. 10, Philadelphia, 1955, J. B. Lippincott Co., chap. 3, pp. 114-126, 159-178, chaps. 13, 17, 21, 24, 25.
8. Emerson, C. P., Jr., and Bragdon, J. S.: Essentials of medicine, ed. 17, Philadelphia, 1955, J. B. Lippincott Co., p. 446.
9. Felter, R. K., West, F., and Zetzsche, L.: Surgical nursing, ed. 6, Philadelphia, 1952, F. A. Davis Co., chaps. 4, 10, unit V, chap. 27, unit IX, chap. 32.
10. Harmer, B., and Henderson, V.: The principles and practice of nursing, New York, 1955, The Macmillan Co., chaps. 26, 29, 31, 37, 39.
11. Holmquist, E. W.: Nursing the adult tracheotomized patient, Amer. J. Nurs. **47:**310-314, 1947.
12. Marten, H., and Ehrlich, H. E.: Nursing care following laryngectomy, Amer. J. Nur. **49:**149-152, 1949.
13. Merrill, V.: Atlas of roentgenographic positions, ed. 3, vol. I, St. Louis, 1967, The C. V. Mosby Co.
14. McClain, M. E., and Gragg, S. H.: Scientific principles in nursing, ed. 5, St. Louis, 1966, The C. V. Mosby Co., chaps. 15, 26, 28, 29.
15. Montag, M. L., and Swenson, R. P. S.: Fundamentals in nursing care, ed. 3, Philadelphia, 1959, W. B. Saunders Co., chaps. 17, 20, 24.

Care of the psychiatric patient

16. Bailly, H.: Nursing mental diseases, New York, 1950, The Macmillan Co.
17. Brownell, K. O.: A textbook of practical nursing, Philadelphia, 1954, W. B. Saunders Co., chap. 18.
18. Cecil, R. L., and Leob, R. K.: A textbook of medicine, Philadelphia, 1955, W. B. Saunders Co., pp. 1656-1683.
19. Fitzsimmon, L.: Textbook for psychiatric attendants, New York, 1947, The Macmillan Co., chaps. 1, 2.
20. Neese, C. C.: Radiographic problems of the mental patient, X-ray Technician **27:**258, 1956.
21. Noyes, A. P., and Haydon, E.: Textbook of psychiatric nursing, New York, 1946, The Macmillan Co.
22. Rhodes, J. M.: Radiological practice with psychiatric patients, X-ray Technician **31:** 256-258, 1959.
23. Schwartz, M. S., and Shockley, E. L.: The nurse and the mental patient, New York, 1956, Russell Sage Foundation.
24. Weiss, M. O.: Attitudes in psychiatric nursing care, New York, 1954, G. P. Putnam's Sons, chaps. 1, 2.

Care of the paralyzed or physically handicapped patient

25. Bierman, W., and Prochozka, A.: Hemiplegia and the nursing care of hemiplegia, Amer. J. Nur. **46:**115-120, 1946.
26. Davis, L.: Christopher's textbook of surgery, Philadelphia, 1956, W. B. Saunders Co., chap. 32.

27. Deaver, G. G., Jerome, M. M., and Taylor, W. E.: Rehabilitation, Amer. J. Nur. **59**:1278-1281, 1959.
28. Grayson, M.: Psychiatric aspects of rehabilitation. J. Nerv. Ment. Dis. **112**:453, 1950.
29. Harmer, B., and Henderson, V.: A textbook of the principles and practices of nursing, New York, 1955, The Macmillan Co., chap. 16.
30. Kessler, H. H.: The principles and practice of rehabilitation. In Bennett, R. L.: Rehabilitation in poliomyelitis, Philadelphia, 1956, Lea & Febiger.
31. Moore, D.: The hemiplegic patient as a person, Public Health Nurs. **40**:511-517, 1948.
32. Morrissey, A. B.: Rehabilitation nursing, New York, 1951, G. P. Putnam's Sons.
33. Terry, F. J., Benz, G. S., Mereness, D., Kleffner, F. R., and Jensen, D. M.: Principles and technics of rehabilitation nursing, St. Louis, 1961, The C. V. Mosby Co., chap. 16.

Care of the patient with a communicable disease
34. A textbook of sterilization, Chicago, 1942, Lakeside Press.
35. Anderson, G. W., and Arnstein, M. G.: Communicable disease control, New York, 1948, The Macmillan Co., part I, pp. 3-147.
36. Benson, M. E.: Handwashing—an important part of medical asepsis, Amer. J. Nurs. **57**:1136, 1957.
37. Brown, A. F.: Medical nursing, ed. 3, Philadelphia, 1957, W. B. Saunders Co., chap. 27.
38. Emerson, C. P., and Bragdon, J. S.: Essentials of medicine, ed. 17, Philadelphia, 1955, J. B. Lippincott Co., chap. 27.
39. Gage, N., London, J. F., and Sider, H. T.: Communicable diseases, ed. 6, Philadelphia, 1951, F. A. Davis Co., unit I.
40. Lynch, T. I.: Communicable disease nursing, ed. 2, St. Louis, 1950, The C. V. Mosby Co.
41. McCulloch, E.: Disinfection and sterilization, ed. 2, Philadelphia, 1945, Lea & Febiger.
42. The control of communicable diseases in man, New York, 1955, American Public Health Association.

Chapter 6

The technician and special patient care— indications for only bedside radiography

The patients referred to in the previous chapter are those whom the x-ray technician may radiograph either at the bedside *or* in the department, depending upon the degree of illness and the stage of convalescence. There are some patients, however, whose condition warrants *only* bedside radiography. These are *some* orthopedic and cardiac patients, the seriously ill patient who is in a respirator, or the patient who is receiving oxygen therapy.

THE ORTHOPEDIC PATIENT
Advantages of portable equipment

Portable x-ray equipment has one real advantage in that it possesses extreme maneuverability. It is possible to lower the portable x-ray tube to floor level and even under the bed to allow shooting toward the ceiling; in fact, radiography of the patient is possible from nearly any conceivable angle. Many times the advantages of maneuverability may well offset the disadvantages due to its limited capacity. The orthopedic patient is usually immobilized by casts, ropes, pulleys, or other orthopedic appliances. In those instances where the patient is *not* completely immobilized by orthopedic apparatus, the part being radiographed can usually *be* immobilized with sandbags. If the technician uses extreme care, the quality of the films produced portably on the orthopedic patient can be as good or better than those produced with high capacity equipment in the main x-ray department.

General considerations in patient care

The approach to the problem, however, must be carefully considered. If the part to be radiographed is thick (lateral films of the hip or spine), use of the grid cassette is indicated. The patient should be advised that his continued treatment and progress are somewhat dependent upon the quality of the film that can be produced to guide his doctor in treatment. The technician should explain to the patient that the equipment being used for his examination is more limited in capacity than that used in the x-ray department and, hence, much is dependent upon the patient's cooperation.

Reporting to the charge nurse and carrying through all her suggestions about safely positioning and immobilizing the patient are essential. These

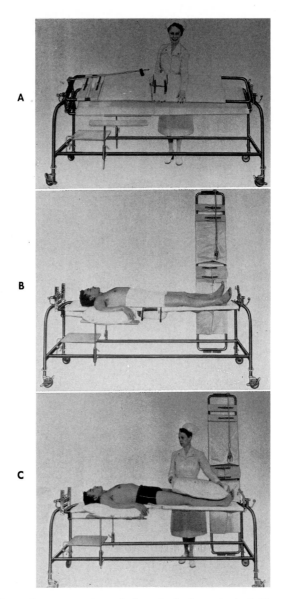

Fig. 6-1. Care of a patient on an orthopedic frame—the Foster bed. **A,** The orthopedic bed, called a Foster frame, consists of a posterior frame on which the patient lies in a supine position and an anterior frame, which is placed on top of him when he is to be turned over. On this frame he lies in the prone position. Both frames can be hyperextended, and traction devices are at either end. **B,** The patient lies on the posterior frame with arms supported by pillows on the arm rests. **C,** The nurse is preparing to turn the patient over. A pillow is placed over the knees to compensate for the lower height of the legs as compared to the chest.

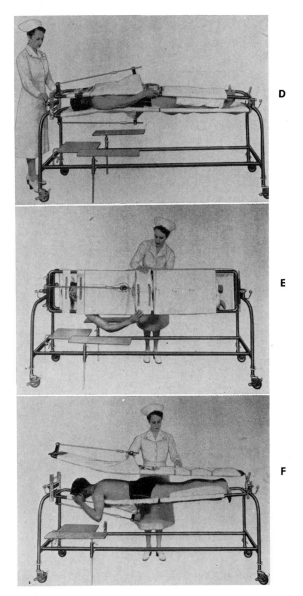

Fig. 6-1, cont'd. D, The anterior frame fits evenly and securely over the body. It is locked into position at each end. **E,** The patient is turned over quickly. Knowledge and skill are required. Some frames require more than one person to operate. The technician should never attempt it alone, however. **F,** With the posterior frame removed, the patient lies prone on the anterior frame. The arm rests can be raised to a comfortable height. A tray of food or reading material can be placed on the adjustable board below so the patient can feed himself, if possible, or read. (Courtesy Gilbert Hyde-Chick Co., Oakland, Calif.)

patients often have an overhead trapeze to grasp in positioning themselves, and they can thereby aid the technician immeasurably. The technician must always take great care to avoid disturbing a patient's traction apparatus. Weights must never be removed under any circumstances. Ropes and pulleys must not be manipulated in any way.

A technician's major responsibility in radiography of this kind is awareness of the patient's complaints and promptness in reporting them to the charge nurse. After a cast has been applied to any part of the body, signs of poor circulation must be observed by *all* members of the medical team who care for the patient. For example, during radiography, a patient in an arm or leg cast might well tell the technician that his toes or fingers tingled, were numb, or were painful. Or, the technician might note a pale or blue color of the extremities distal to the cast. These are danger signs and should always be reported promptly to the charge nurse at the completion of the film.

The orthopedic frame

Occasionally the technician will be asked to take an x-ray picture of a patient on an orthopedic frame. There are several kinds—Bradford, Stryker, and Foster frames, and others, but all accomplish the same purpose—immobilizing or hyperextending a patient so that his body alignment is not interferred with, yet at the same time simplifying turning and caring for him (Fig. 6-1). There is an anterior and a posterior frame, each padded and covered, supported on a movable frame cart. The patient lies on his back on the posterior frame and when he must be turned over, the anterior frame is placed over him and locked into position over his face and body. The frame is turned 180 degrees so that the patient is lying on his face on the anterior frame. This facilitates nursing care, allows the patient perhaps to read or feed himself, and also makes it *safe* to turn him. The frame is most often used for patients with spinal cord injuries or paraplegia. In these conditions it is important that proper body alignment be maintained, since torsion of any part of the spine could result in permanent cord injury and permanent paralysis. Occasionally a surgical patient will be placed on the frame to allow for free drainage of a wound.

If a patient must be turned on his face or his back to have a portable x-ray film taken, the technician must never, under any circumstances, attempt this maneuver alone. A nurse *must* supervise the turning of the patient, and at least two people must be present to carry out the procedure correctly and safely. Let us assume that the physician has ordered a posteroanterior film of the lumbar spine for a patient on such a frame. The patient will probably be in the supine position to begin with and his neck movement limited so that it is impossible to position a cassette underneath the spine area. The cassette could conceivably be placed under the frame, but portions of the apparatus would then appear on the film and might block out the area in which some pathology was suspected. The technician should enlist the aid of a nurse from the station. The grid cassette should be positioned properly over the patient's abdomen and pelvic areas so as to include those vertebrae which are to be radiographed. The nurse would then slip down the top frame so that it fits over the patient and the cassette and lock it into position. The patient then could be rotated to the prone position so that he would be lying on his stomach on the cassette. After removing the posterior frame, the x-ray tube would be brought into position and the exposure made. Upon completion of the exposure, the frame would be reattached and locked, the patient rotated to the supine position and the anterior frame and cassette removed, thereby obtaining a posteroanterior view of the part in question. If the anteroposterior view is preferred, the radiograph could be obtained by using the same general procedure as outlined, with one exception; the patient would start in the prone position and the cassette would be placed on his back before attaching the frame and rotating him into the anteroposterior position. If the cassette can be slipped under his neck or spine to take the film, without turning

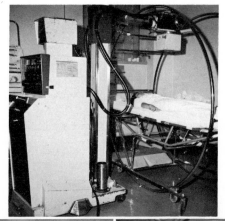

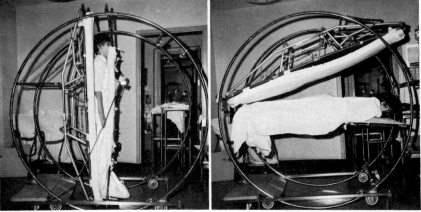

Fig. 6-2. The new circular bed often used in lieu of the orthopedic frame described in Fig. 6-1.

him over, the nurse should be the one to assume the responsibility for placing the cassette.

These patients are very nervous and apprehensive about their existence on the frame. The frame is narrow which gives the patient the feeling of not being very stable. He is constantly fearful that he will fall off the frame when he is turned. Naturally this will not happen if he is turned in the proper way. However, if the technician is wide-eyed or if she shows signs of fear—like surprise or breathlessness—it will only increase the patient's anxiety. It is vital that the medical team be calm, matter-of-fact, and yet aware of the potential hazards when caring for these patients.

A comparatively recent development, the CircOlectric bed, has come into general use in place of the orthopedic frame (Fig. 6-2). The CircOlectric bed allows for vertical turning. Unassisted, the nurse can change a patient's position, but more important is the fact that the patient can position himself with the use of the electrical controls. The CircOlectric bed is very maneuverable, and it is possible for the radiologic technologist to obtain the necessary films on patients occupying this kind of an orthopedic device with less difficulty than might be true if the patient was in one of the other types of previously described orthopedic frames.

THE CRITICALLY ILL PATIENT
Radiographic technique necessary

The critically ill patient will necessarily present many special radiographic problems if his physician believes that he cannot be moved to the main x-ray department. Basically, however, all patients who are critically ill will have one common problem—inability to cooperate in stopping voluntary or involuntary motion. Radiography of these patients, regardless of the type of film requested, will always necessitate using the x-ray equipment at its higher kilovoltage capacities and at the maximum milliampere capacity in order to ensure the fastest possible exposure time.

It might be well for the student technician to review the unsharpness formula which incorporates the factors that affect detail. Such review should establish firmly in mind the exact effect of exposure time and motion on detail in a radiograph. It must be remembered that motion affects detail on a radiograph to a greater extent than any other single factor. Bearing this in mind, several things can be done when it is necessary to obtain the maximum detail on the films of this type of patient. Two possibilities have been enumerated which will enable the technician to shorten the exposure time on a radiograph, namely, using the equipment at its higher capacity in both milliamperage and voltage. If one finds that proper adjustment of kilovoltage and milliamperage would still leave an opportunity, in so far as timer capacity is concerned, to obtain a shorter exposure time, the next step would be to shorten the focal film distance. This *is* contrary to good radiographic practice, since a short focal film distance causes a loss of detail. However, the gain possible with this type of compromise may permit one to shorten the exposure time. Again, referring to the unsharpness formula, one finds that the juggling of these factors is nearly always in favor of a short exposure time in order to obtain the best detail.

In making radiographs on this type of patient, one should take full advantage of the maneuverability of portable x-ray equipment. In ordinary radiographic practice, the patient is usually positioned for certain types of projections because *he* is more maneuverable than the x-ray equipment. For portable radiography, a departure from this standard should be considered wherever possible in order to arrive at a result which involves as little handling of the patient as possible and utilizes the maneuverability of the equipment instead.

The decision about what to do on the portable x-ray examination rests with the technician, and the success of the examination is often the result of experience. The technician should bear in mind how an examination is ordinarily done in the main x-ray department, then arrive at a decision as to what departure from the routine method can best be used when the condition of the patient dictates a change from normal procedure.

An example may be the patient for whom a lateral skull film is ordered to be taken with portable x-ray equipment. There will be a departure from the normal procedure, which is to have the patient in a semiprone, oblique position with the skull in the lateral position. In doing this examination portably, it would be best to have the patient remain supine on the hospital bed, to build up the head with pillows and to utilize the maneuverability of the tube by bringing it to bed level and projecting the central beam across the bed to obtain the radiograph. A short focal film distance could be used to obtain an extremely short exposure time. If the patient is suffering from a skull injury, he may be comatose or unconscious and unable to cooperate at all. Although the results of radiography made with short focal film distance are going to be magnified and distorted, the advantage gained by short exposure time would probably disclose fracture lines to better advantage than if a normal focal film distance had been used with the resulting longer exposure time.

A plywood box large enough for holding a cassette is also helpful in radiography of the critically ill patient, especially one requiring anteroposterior chest films. If the patient is so ill that any exertion on his part will result in increased chest and lung motion, it is probably best to film him in the supine position. In many instances the hospital bed will be cranked up slightly to bring the patient into a reclining position rather than a completely supine position in order to ease his respiration. The best procedure would be to slide the cassette in the box under the patient's chest, compensate for angulation of the bed with angulation of the tube in order to maintain a vertical relationship between the film and the tube, and then make the exposure, utilizing a short focal film distance to obtain the fastest possible exposure time. If such a box is not used, the patient, when reclining on the cassette, will tend to throw either one side or the other of the screens in the cassette out of contact unless, by sheer accident, the weight of the patient is very evenly distributed. The result will be a fuzzy chest film with a lack of detail on one section of the film which could be confused with some types of pathology. Incorporating the use of the box described will ensure that the screens of the cassette inserted in such a box and placed under the patient will maintain equal contact. A box of this nature should be used in all portable x-ray work whenever the weight of the patient will be on the cassette.

THE CARDIAC PATIENT

A comparatively high percentage of portable x-rays requested in any hospital will be for the patient with heart disease. An important factor in the care of the acutely ill cardiac patient is rest, physical and mental rest. Even moving him from the bed to a litter to the x-ray department may be out of the question, since it might jeopardize his recovery. The patient may have arteriosclerotic heart disease, such as coronary thrombosis, in which the blood vessels have become narrowed due to the normal degenerative process of aging. He may have an inflammatory disease like rheumatic fever or endocarditis. He may have hypertensive heart disease or one of many other diseases of the heart.

The technician, on entering the patient's room, may easily be deceived as to the condition of the patient. He may appear to be resting comfortably and show little evidence of the seriousness of his condition. In fact, the technician may think there is no indication for portable radiography. However, it must be remembered that a cardiac patient may be existing with very little vital reserve. The maneuvering of the patient or his bed might exhaust this reserve and have serious consequences. Therefore, it is imperative that the technician solicit the cooperation of the nurse in handling this type of patient, since the nurse will be more familiar with the patient's condition and will advise the technician of the limitations on the patient's movement and activity. Patients are classified according to the acuteness of their particular disease, and this in turn determines the amount of activity which they can safely tolerate. Some can roll over while the cassette is placed in position. Others can do nothing. They cannot raise their heads or reach for a glass of water. When the technician is working with these patients, the charge nurse will send one or more of her staff members to help.

The technician should be aware of why the examination is being requested. If congestion of the chest is suspected, then the procedure outlined in the previous section should be followed for taking the chest film. However, if the x-ray film is being made to determine heart size, it may be necessary to maintain a longer focal film distance than normal in order to obtain a less distorted heart size. It will be impossible with portable x-ray equipment to obtain a chest film for heart size with the patient supine, since inadequate focal film distance with resulting distortion would result. Therefore, it will require that the patient be seated on the edge of the bed for a conventional upright film of the chest at a 6-foot distance. This position would require permission of the doctor.

Special care must be taken to move quietly and with assurance. Careful explanation about what is to be done is necessary so as not to frighten or disturb the patient or to disrupt in any way the plan of mental and physical rest made for him by the medical team.

THE PATIENT RECEIVING OXYGEN THERAPY

Every living person and thing needs oxygen to grow and keep alive, but in certain illnesses and conditions, some patients require more oxygen than the air contains. Oxygen accounts for about 20.9% of atmospheric air, nitrogen 79.04%, and carbon dioxide 0.3%. When this amount of oxygen, however, is not enough to supply the body needs, the patient has a dusky blue color, called cyanosis, which is most apparent in the lips and nails. Too, he usually shows some signs of dyspnea or labored breathing. This increased demand for oxygen is characteristic in some lung conditions, such as pneumonia or asthma, and in certain types of heart disease. Oxygen is given during most operations and is frequently used after others, especially operations on the chest.

The three most common ways to give oxygen to a patient are by use of (1) the oxygen tent, in which the patient's head or entire body is inside a transparent canopy (Fig. 6-3); (2) the mask, which fits either over the patient's nose

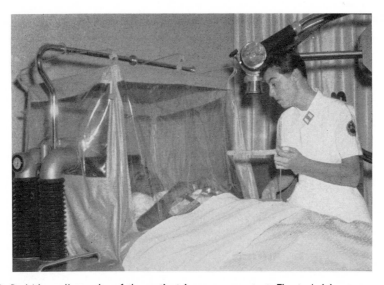

Fig. 6-3. Bedside radiography of the patient in an oxygen tent. The technician arranges for all technical factors for the portable machine and even positions the patient before the nurse is asked to turn off the oxygen and remove the patient from the tent. Because of possible explosion hazards in an area of oxygen, all possible sources of friction are eliminated. Note the special signal bell instead of the usual type. Electrical and x-ray machines must be checked for good working order.

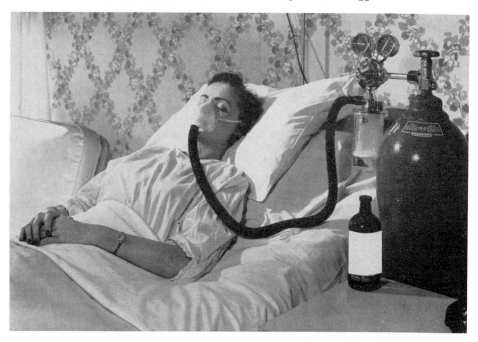

Fig. 6-4. A patient receiving oxygen therapy by the oronasal type mask. The amount of oxygen the patient receives is controlled by the device above the bottle. Oxygen bubbles into the bottle of water from the tank for humidification before it is breathed by the patient. (Courtesy the National Cylinder Gas Co., Chicago, Ill.)

or over both his nose and mouth (Fig. 6-4); and (3) the nasal catheter or tube which is inserted into the nasal passage (Fig. 6-5). The choice of any of the methods is dependent on the patient's condition, his restlessness, age, and other factors. The nasal method is most efficient in that little oxygen is wasted in the administration. The tent method is least efficient, in that, despite the tent being closed and tucked under the mattress, some oxygen is bound to escape. On the other hand, it is more comfortable. The mask method is fairly efficient but is somewhat irritating to the patient's face.

Most often oxygen is directed to the tent, mask, or catheter from a tank or cylinder of compressed oxygen, through a regulator which permits the rate of flow to be controlled as prescribed by the doctor. Some hospitals now have oxygen piped into the patients' rooms, and the tubing from the tent, mask, or catheter is attached to the regulator and then directly to the wall outlet of oxygen.

Care of these patients is very specific and detailed, and while it is not the responsibility of the technician to care for the patient, awareness of some hazards involved in oxygen therapy is essential. Oxygen is not combustible but is a violent supporter of combustion. Materials which burn slowly in atmospheric air flare up and are consumed with great rapidity in an atmosphere rich in oxygen. Therefore, it is extremely important to prevent all sources of ignition

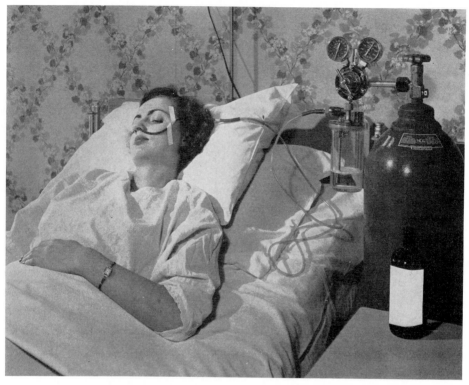

Fig. 6-5. A patient receiving oxygen therapy by nasal catheter. While this is the most efficient method of giving oxygen therapy with little loss of oxygen, it can be used in only selected cases, where the age or condition of the patient will not be a factor in the accidental removal of the tube. (Courtesy the National Cylinder Gas Co., Chicago, Ill.)

from coming in close proximity to oxygen. These sources are oily fingers, alcohol, call bells, electric suction machines, x-ray machines, etc. Any of these could produce a spark, which would result in fire when oxygen is being administered to a patient. Therefore, when a portable x-ray is to be made, the charge nurse will see that a nurse accompanies the technician to the patient's room. The *nurse* temporarily will remove the tent or mask from the patient and turn off the oxygen. If the patient is receiving oxygen by nasal catheter, the catheter is left in place and the oxygen supply turned off while the x-ray is being taken.

Most frequently, the examination requested will be a chest plate which will have to be obtained with the best possible exposure speed because of the patient's critical condition. Occasionally the attending physician may believe that the patient in a tent cannot be without oxygen. With the assistance of the nurse, the tent would then be draped around the patient's head, leaving the chest area free for the radiographic examination. It may be possible, however, to take the patient completely out of the tent for a short period of time. If so, all preparations for the examination should be made while the patient is still in the tent. Patients re-

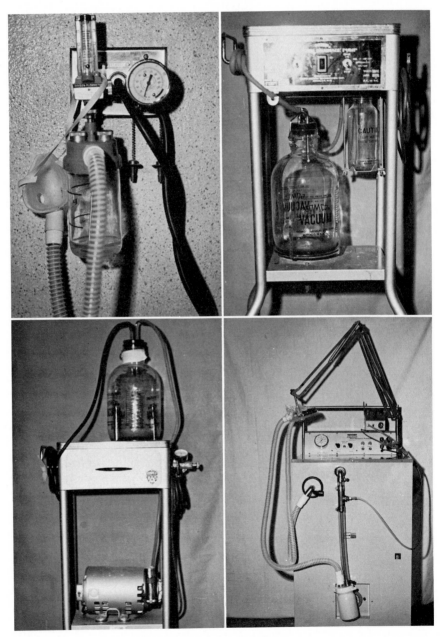

Fig. 6-6. Various methods of aiding respiration can be handled by apparatus shown in these illustrations.

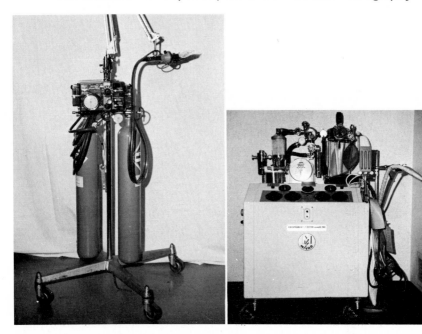

Fig. 6-6, cont'd. For legend see opposite page.

quiring oxygen therapy generally are quite sick, and to be cut off from the oxygen supply, even for a short period, not only makes them more fearful and apprehensive but also retards their progress. Therefore, the technician should adjust the machine and have it all ready before the oxygen is turned off, thus decreasing the amount of time the patient is without oxygen. This includes placing the cassette under him, setting the exposure factors on the x-ray control, instructing the patient as to what is expected of him, if he is in condition to be at all cooperative, and having all arrangements for the radiograph made. Then the only thing necessary when the patient is removed from the tent is to place the tube over the cassette and the patient and immediately make the exposure.

REFERENCES

The orthopedic patient

1. Davis, L.: Christopher's textbook of surgery, Philadelphia, 1956, W. B. Saunders Co., chap. 28.
2. Eliason, E., Ferguson, L. K., and Sholtis, L.: Surgical nursing, ed. 10, Philadelphia, 1955, J. B. Lippincott Co., chaps. 24, 25.
3. Harmer, B., and Henderson, V.: Textbook of the principles and practice of nursing, New York, 1955, The Macmillan Co., chap. 42.
4. Larson, C. B., and Gould, M.: Calderwood's orthopedic nursing, ed. 6, St. Louis, 1965, The C. V. Mosby Co., units II, XII, XIII.
5. Mella, M.: The mental rehabilitation of patients with spinal cord injuries, Amer. J. Nurs. 45:370-373, 1945.
6. Pielock, C. R., and Sagath, E. E.: Spinal cord injuries and the Stryker frame, Amer. J. Nurs. 45:360-370, 1945.

7. Skinner, G.: Nursing care of a patient on a Stryker frame, Amer. J. Nurs. **46**:288-292, 1946.
8. Stafford, E. S., and Diller, D.: Textbook of surgery for nurses. Philadelphia, 1954, W. B. Saunders Co., chap. 44.

The patient in a respirator

9. Brown, A. F.: Medical nursing, Philadelphia, 1957, W. B. Saunders Co., pp. 138-144.
10. Harmer, B., and Henderson, V.: Textbook of principles and practice of nursing, New York, 1955, The Macmillan Co., chap. 27.
11. Hull, E., and Perrodin, C.: Medical nursing, Philadelphia, 1952, F. A. Davis Co., pp. 150-163.
12. Isolation techniques and nursing care in poliomyelitis, New York, 1952, National Foundation for Infantile Paralysis.
13. Kottke, F. J., and Kubicek, W. G.: The patient with bulbar-respiratory poliomyelitis, Amer. J. Nurs. **49**:374-377, 1949.
14. Larson, C. B., and Gould, M.: Calderwood's orthopedic nursing, ed. 6, St. Louis, 1965, The C. V. Mosby Co., unit VIII.
15. Nursing for the poliomyelitis patient, New York, 1948. Prepared and published by the Joint Orthopedic Nursing Advisory Service of the NOPHN and the NLNE, 1790 Broadway, New York.
16. Parisi, C.: The patient in a respirator, Amer. J. Nurs. **51**:360-363, 1951.
17. Steigman, A. J., and Rumph, P. H.: Teh positive-pressure dome, Amer. J. Nurs. **52**:311-312, 1952.

The cardiac patient

18. Brown, A. F.: Medical nursing, ed. 3, Philadelphia, 1957, W. B. Saunders Co., chap. 13.
19. Cecil, R. L., and Loeb, R. F.: A textbook of medicine, Philadelphia, 1955, W. B. Saunders Co., pp. 1230-1374.
20. Crowley, E. M.: Convalescent care in heart disease, Amer. J. Nurs. **44**:1124-1128, 1944.
21. Emerson, C. P., and Bragdon, J. S.: Essentials of medicine, ed. 17, Philadelphia, 1955, J. B. Lippincott Co., chap. 13.
22. Goldsmith, M. G.: Rheumatic heart disease in children, Public Health Nurs. **32**:711-714, 1940.
23. Hull, E., and Perrodin, C.: Medical nursing, Philadelphia, 1952, W. A. Davis Co., unit III.
24. Jayne, M.: Nursing care of the acutely ill cardiac patient, Amer. J. Nurs. **38**:1325, 1938.
25. Ravin, A., and Ravin, R. R.: The acutely ill cardiac patient, Amer. J. Nurs. **38**:1318-1325, 1938.
26. Taylor, A.: Comforts for the cardiac patient, Amer. J. Nurs. **38**:768, 1938.

The patient receiving oxygen therapy

27. Brown, A. F.: Medical nursing, Philadelphia, 1957, W. B. Saunders Co., pp. 109-138.
28. Eliason, E., Ferguson, L. K., and Sholtis, L.: Surgical nursing, Philadelphia, 1955, J. B. Lippincott Co., pp. 178-185.
29. Emerson, C. P., and Bragdon, J. S.: Essentials of medicine, ed. 17, Philadelphia, 1955, J. B. Lippincott Co., pp. 120-126.
30. Harmer, B., and Henderson, V.: Textbook of the principles and practice of nursing, New York, 1955, The Macmillan Co., chap. 27.
31. Hull, E., and Perrodin, C.: Medical nursing, Philadelphia, 1952, Administration of oxygen, carbon dioxide and helium, F. A. Davis Co., pp. 139-150.
32. Livingstone, H. M.: Safety measures in oxygen therapy, Inhalation Therapy Bulletin, vol. 1, no. 2, 1950.
33. Livingstone, H. M.: Nursing care in oxygen therapy, Amer. J. Nurs. **55**:65, 1955.
34. Montag, M. L., and Swenson, R. P. S.: Fundamentals in nursing care, ed. 3, Philadelphia, 1959, W. B. Saunders Co., chap. 23.
35. Oxygen therapy handbook, New York, 1957, The Linde Air Products Co.

Chapter 7

The patient and diagnostic examinations

GASTROINTESTINAL EXAMINATION
Intrinsic and extrinsic disease

The gastrointestinal series of examinations include those which are required for the study of the esophagus, stomach, and small bowel. Fluoroscopy may be carried on with the aim of discovering either an intrinsic or extrinsic disease. In the case of the esophagus, intrinsic diseases are those that involve the esophagus itself, such as cancer, fistulas (holes or openings into tissue), atresias (strictures). Extrinsic disease is that which involves an area surrounding the esophagus and causes displacement or invasion of it. The esophagus also serves as a landmark for the study of cardiac enlargement and thyroid tumors. The patient with esophageal disease may have pain, difficulty in swallowing, called dysphagia, or there may be bleeding.

Examination of the stomach is also carried on for the purpose of discovering intrinsic or extrinsic disease. The intrinsic diseases which commonly involve the stomach are the various malignancies, benign tumors, and ulcers. Extrinsic disease is any disease or enlargement of organs in the surrounding area which might cause encroachment upon or displacement of the stomach. Cysts, abscesses, diaphragmatic hernias, and liver enlargement are examples of extrinsic disease. A patient with suspected involvement of the stomach frequently has had loss of appetite (anorexia) and therefore appears pale and thin. He may have been having pain or bleeding, the blood being noticed in either an emesis or in tarry stools. Studies of the small bowel are made with the view of discovering anything that may be causing obstruction of it either through disease of the small bowel itself or encroachment of a surrounding area.

Preparation of the patient

Preparation of the patient for "G.I. series" usually begins 12 to 14 hours before the actual examination is done. The patient is restricted to a light meal the previous evening. He is given nothing by mouth, fluid or otherwise, after eight o'clock in the evening, and if possible, oral medication should be stopped. The patient then reports to the x-ray department for the examination at eight o'clock in the morning of the following day. In most instances the fluoroscopy and films of a gastrointestinal series can be completed in approximately 15 minutes unless the disease dictates some special techniques.

119

In the case of small bowel studies, however, it would be necessary to have follow-up x-ray films for several succeeding hours following the original fluoroscopic examination, hence the name "series." As this usually involves withholding food or drink from the patient, it is necessary that the technician clearly explain this to the charge nurse on the station. If the patient is not hospitalized and is an outpatient, he should be told to report back to the x-ray department at stated intervals throughout the day and should be given written instructions that nothing may be taken by mouth until such time as the radiologist has indicated the completion of the examination.

Explanation to the patient

Because of the very nature of the fluoroscopic examination, a thorough explanation to the patient is essential. Darkness is not to be feared if it is understood and explained in advance. However, it is most distressing for a patient to undergo fluoroscopic examination if the technician merely assumes that he knows the lights will be off. The patient should be told that the sounds of the machine are due to repeated spot films during the examination. He should know that the table will be tilted repeatedly and he should be assured that he will be held firmly during the tilting. The reason that the doctor and technicians are wearing gloves and aprons should be explained to the patient. The radiologist should be introduced to the patient upon entering the room. The patient should know that the doctor will be palpating and pushing on the abdomen during the examination.

The administration of the barium sulfate should be explained. For oral ingestion it should be made as palatable as possible and shown to the patient while the lights are on so he can see what it looks like and how much he is expected to drink. He should be told to drink it only upon the radiologist's request. Because is can be constipating if not evacuated, the patient is usually given or told to take an ounce of milk of magnesia following oral ingestion and then told to watch for the barium in his stools within the next day or so.

The development of the image intensifier has helped to solve many problems in connection with fluoroscopic examinations. When this instrument is used, fluoroscopic examinations can be carried out without completely darkening the room. The many advantages of this unit are explained in Chapter 9. Carrying on a fluoroscopic examination in a room with subdued light rather than total darkness is reassuring to the patient.

Positioning of the patient

In most departments the radiologist carries on work in two fluoroscopic rooms simultaneously. The radiologist fluoroscopes a patient in one room while the technician is taking films of the patient on whom he has completed fluoroscopy in another room.

There are four possible positions involved in taking films following the fluoroscopy. The posteroanterior position with the patient prone is used, since it causes the stomach to spread out and gives a good view of the duodenal loop. The anteroposterior position with the patient supine has only one purpose generally—and that is to give an adequate view of the distended fundus filled with barium and the air-filled antrum. The oblique positions are taken to give different views of the stomach wall, while the lateral position is important in displacement of various kinds and for the best viewing of the duodenojejunal junction.

After completing the films, the technician should assist the patient from the table and return him to the dressing room area. The technician should then prepare the room for another patient and prepare the patient for the forthcoming examination.

COLON EXAMINATION
Diseases of the colon

In x-ray vernacular, colon studies are usually called barium enemas and/or air contrast enemas. The study is a combination of fluoroscopy by the radiologist and the taking of films by the x-ray technician. The colon is one of the most common sites of malignancy, but it is also a site where a high percentage of cures is effected. In addition, this examination will disclose what many believe to be premalignant lesions, small nodules called "polyps." It may also demonstrate inflammatory lesions such as tuberculosis, diverticulitis, or colitis.

The patient with colon disease frequently complains of a change in bowel habits—either constipation or diarrhea. He may have noticed blood in his stools, in which case it is *not* dark, tarry, and digested blood indicative of disease higher up in the gastrointestinal tract, but rather it is fresh and red. He may also have had pain or weight loss.

Preparation of the patient

An empty colon, like any other hollow organ with muscular walls, will not cast a separate shadow on a film. When filled with barium or air it can be outlined. Therefore, proper and thorough patient preparation is extremely important so that the colon will be cleared of all fecal material and flatus. The shadows of density that they cause under fluoroscopy could make difficult or confuse the diagnosis of the radiologist. After evacuation of barium, enough usually remains to show the pattern of the mucosa or lining. Frequently air is injected after the barium has been expelled, and thus a double contrast of barium and air may outline polyps which might otherwise be missed.

There is some conflict as to what is the best method for preparing a patient for barium enema series. However, it is generally agreed that the patient should have no food after the evening meal. He should have enemas, either tap water, soap suds, or salt water, until clear the evening prior to the examination. In many instances, 2 ounces of castor oil are recommended several hours prior to the examination. Enemas are frequently ordered in the morning again. Preparation for air contrast enema is similar to that for the regular barium enema with the exception that a low residue diet for several days prior to the examination is helpful. The technical and nursing staffs must be scrupulous in their preparation of the patient as an aid toward a successful examination.

Explanation to the patient

A patient who is to receive a barium enema should have a very thorough explanation of the whole procedure, not only to lessen his fears and apprehensions but also to enable him to cooperate more fully with the radiologist and technician.

The darkened room, the appearance of the doctor, and the mechanics of the enema administration should be explained. It is essential to his well-being that he should be told about the hard table, the tube insertion, and how much fluid he will have to take and keep from expelling. It is also wise to tell him that he will be asked to turn back and forth frequently. In view of the darkness and narrow table, he will need to know that the technician is ready to assist and to protect him from injury.

He should know that the doctor will direct the flow of the barium solution by saying "Off" and "On" to the technician. On some occasions a patient attempts to get "off" the table thinking the radiologist is speaking to *him*. He should understand that he will have repeated films, possibly further barium injection and/or air injection, and that there will be need for evacuation after each.

The barium enema

Necessary equipment.

1. *The standard.* The standard should have a broad base so that it will not upset easily, and its height should be easily adjustable. The newer x-ray tables have these directly attached.

2. *Enema can.* A large can holding up to 2 quarts is essential. It is annoying to have to stop in the middle of a fluoroscopic examination to have the can refilled. There is always the possibility of air getting into the tubing before more barium can be added, creating an air lock and preventing the flow of barium. There should be a hole in the top of the can to hang it to the stand. Using a piece of string is unsatisfactory since it may break and the falling can will flood the table, the patient, and the room.

3. *Tubing and glass adapters.* The harder rubber tubing is much better than softer kinds, since the latter kinks easily, thus stopping the flow of barium. The tubing should be long enough to allow the enema can to be raised to the proper height but not so long that it gets in the way of the patient's legs as he is turning.

4. *Clamp.* A good clamp that will completely stop the flow of barium into the tube is one that is easily opened and closed. It is inexcusable to find the colon already half filled with barium when one starts the fluoroscopic examina-

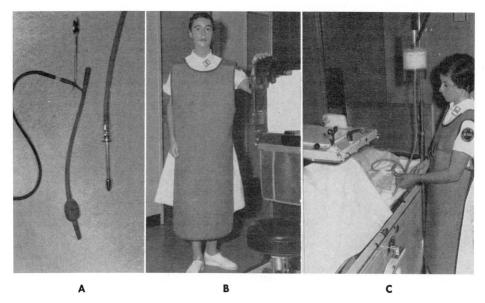

A   **B**   **C**

Fig. 7-1. Colon examination. **A,** Two barium enema tips in use are the Bardex, similar to the urinary retention catheter, only larger, and the metal Carmen tip. **B,** A technician is protected from over-radiation by the leaded apron worn during fluoroscopy. The physician will wear an apron and also protective gloves. The x-ray–sensitive badge on the technician's collar will show whether the amount of radiation the technician receives in a given time is within safe limits. **C,** Adequately protected and covered, the patient is in position for receiving a barium enema. The technician will clamp off the flow of barium at the radiologist's signal.

tion simply because a weak clamp failed to completely close off the flow. Similarly, the flow must be stopped quickly to obtain spot films.

5. *Enema tip* (Fig. 7-1, *A*). The *Carmen tip* is a metal tip, generally used for most patients. It is entirely safe and comfortable if inserted correctly. The *rubber rectal tube,* used in many hospitals for routine enemas, is quite satisfactory and comes in several sizes. It follows the curve of the rectum and causes no discomfort. After repeated boiling, which will make it too soft to insert, it should be discarded. When a patient is old or very ill and there is danger of expelling the barium, a *Bardex tube* with inflatable bag can be used. This is similar to the urinary retention catheter described previously except that it is longer and larger. The Bardex tube is used also in giving a barium enema to a patient with a colostomy.

6. *Air injection apparatus.* A special tube with inflatable bag is made to use in air injections.

7. *Lubricant.* Petrolatum should not be used as a lubricant, since it weakens the rubber. A nonoily lubricant, such as KY, is more expensive but more satisfactory.

8. *Pitcher.* The *pitcher* should be sufficiently large to mix enough barium solution for a full enema.

9. *Long-handled spoon.* The spoon is necessary for stirring the barium mixture.

10. *Thermometer.* Although not routinely used in some departments, it is wise to use a thermometer to test the water temperature before mixing.

Preparation of the barium solution. The barium and water should never be mixed in the enema can, since some lumps may not dissolve and will clog the tubing during the procedure. A mixture of pastelike consistency can be made and mixed with warm water just prior to the enema administration. If prepared sooner, the barium can separate out and will settle on the bottom and in the tube. Care should be taken to have the solution warm—not hot or cold. A small amount can be poured over the inner surface of the wrist to test the temperature. Ideally, it should be tested with a thermometer at a reading between 100° and 105° F. The introduction of cold or hot solutions can be both uncomfortable and dangerous to the patient.

Insertion of the tip (Fig. 7-1, *C*).

1. The patient should be made as comfortable as possible on the table. Great care should be taken to provide for his privacy, keeping doors closed, and exposing and uncovering him only as necessary. He should be turned on his left side, his back to the technician and with both knees flexed.

2. The technician will probably want to wear rubber gloves; in this case to keep the hands from becoming soiled, *not* because it is a sterile procedure.

3. The barium should be allowed to run to the tip, then clamped off, thus expelling air in the tubing before its insertion.

4. Male technicians should introduce the tip in male patients only; female patients should be attended by female technicians.

5. In order to facilitate insertion, several steps are recommended: (a) The enema tip should be well lubricated. (b) The upper buttocks is grasped with one hand and raised to expose and open the anus. (c) The patient is told to relax and to breathe deeply through his mouth. (d) Care should be taken to introduce the tip gently and slowly, especially if the patient has hemorrhoids. (e) The tip is inserted 1 to 2 inches toward the umbilicus, at which time it should be directed back to the sacrum, for a total of 4 to 6 inches. It thus follows the natural curve of the rectum.

6. The patient can then be turned on his back with the tube in place. The clamp is kept tight until the radiologist is ready to do the examination.

7. The can should be elevated 18 to 24 inches above the table level for enema administration.

8. The technician may have to hold the tube in place at the anal outlet if the patient attempts to expel it.

Administration of the barium enema. The patient is examined under fluoroscopy in the darkened room while the barium is being injected. The patient is asked to turn from side to side to separate those parts of the colon which overlap and hide each other. Often a second fluoroscopic examination is done after evacuation to clear up any difficulty in viewing. During the administration of the barium, the abdominal muscles are often contracted and the colon cannot be palpated for a mass or for movement. After evacuation the abdomen becomes soft, and palpation is much more satisfactory.

Spot films are often taken of various areas with the patient so turned as to show that part to the best advantage. The barium is turned off during this interval. Often an oblique film is taken with the patient turned partly on the left side to obtain a view of the sigmoid and descending colon, as soon as these parts have been filled with barium. The barium is again turned off during this period so that the remainder of the colon is not filled with barium, because it may hide the part being examined.

A large film is usually taken after the whole colon is filled with barium. If the barium outlines the appendix or the terminal ileum, one can be sure that the colon has been filled. Often because of the overlapping at the flexures of the descending colon and sigmoid, some of these structures are not visualized on this film. If a fluoroscopic examination were not also done, it would be impossible to say that there were no disease in the overlapped parts (Fig. 7-2).

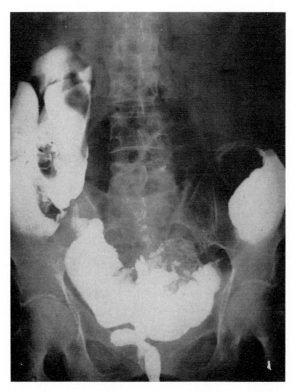

Fig. 7-2. Barium enema.

A postevacuation film is always taken and the pattern of the mucous lining of the colon is usually well outlined.

When an air injection is desired, it should be done by the radiologist after the postevacuation film. This is done under fluoroscopic control, since it is possible to inject too much air, thus causing discomfort or rupture of the colon. Another large film is then taken, using less exposure, because of the air in the bowel.

After completion of the examination, the technician should always assist the patient from the table to the bathroom and see that toilet tissue is handy and that the patient is not left alone if he is weakened due to the procedure. It should be made clear to him when he can eat, so that he is not left weak and hungry any longer than necessary.

The colostomy patient. In giving a barium enema to a patient with a colostomy, the procedure is very similar to that previously described. If the patient has a dressing over the colostomy, it should be removed and discarded in newspapers. Clean rubber gloves may be worn by the technician. A well-lubricated Bardex catheter is used for insertion. The patient should lie on his back during the insertion of the tube and insufflation of the balloon. Due to the smaller bowel capacity, less barium fluid will be necessary. When the patient is ready for evacuation, the Bardex catheter may be left in place until the patient is in the lavatory. He may be seated on the toilet and, using two curved basins interchangeably, can alternately fill the basins with barium and empty them into the toilet. At the end of the procedure, if he is a hospital patient, a large clean pad may be placed over the colostomy as a temporary dressing and the station charge nurse informed of his need for a dressing to provide better protection. If he is an outpatient, he should be supplied with whatever dressings he usually uses.

Care of the equipment. Any barium remaining in the can should be discarded in a toilet or hopper—not a sink, both for aesthetic reasons and because it will plug the drain. The whole enema apparatus should be first rinsed and then scrubbed with hot soapy solution inside and out. Remember that no amount of disinfecting or sterilizing can reach an area covered with feces or any organic material. After washing, the can and tips can be boiled or disinfected in the department or sent to the central supply room to be cared for. Tubing and tips should be boiled for 5 minutes.

The table should be washed off well with soap and water or a disinfectant, and the lavatory should be checked for cleanliness before another patient is admitted. The technician must be scrupulous in her own handwashing.

As mentioned in a previous chapter, the use of disposable material is now a factor in barium enema examinations. Many radiologists prefer to use the prepared barium enema kits with the disposable unit including a bag, the barium, tubing, and an enema tip, all of which can be disposed of following the examination. This unquestionably saves time and permits standardization. Many radiologists, however, believe that the method described is preferable.

BILIARY TRACT EXAMINATION
Cholecystography

General considerations. X-ray examination of the gallbladder is another of the many examinations done in the x-ray department which involves a considerable amount of patient preparation prior to the examination and patient care during the examination. The roentgenographic examination of the gallbladder is made possible by the use of various opaque dyes which, when given either by mouth or intravenously, will enter the liver. From the hepatic cells the contrast substance is excreted with the bile and conveyed to the gallbladder. When the contrast substance is given orally, it is absorbed through the intestinal mucosa by the portal blood stream and enters the liver through the portal vein. When it is given intravenously, the dye is carried through the circulatory system and into the liver through the hepatic artery.

This method of examining the gallbladder was developed by Drs. Graham, Cole, and Copher in 1924. Until the Graham-Cole test had been originated, the only method of examining the gallbladder radiographically was by routine film of the *area*. It was possible to demonstrate stones in the gallbladder area only if they were of the opaque type, not the radiolucent type. However, at that time there was no assurances that the calcifications observed were actually within the limits of the gallbladder. X-ray technique plus the use of opaque dyes now make it possible to determine with reasonable accuracy the presence of either the radiolucent type of stone or the opaque type of stone in the gallbladder. The radiopaque type also permits determination of a *functioning* gallbladder. In recent years it has become possible to detect the presence of stones in the biliary ducts by the use of intravenous opaque dyes.

Preparation of the patient. When a request is made for a gallbladder examination (commonly called a cholecystogram), it is extremely important that an accurate patient history is available to the radiologist. The history should include any report of a previous x-ray examination of the digestive tract, whether the patient is jaundiced, and whether he has a record of unusual drug allergies. Any medication which might affect the usual function of the liver, the gallbladder, or the gastrointestinal tract should be discontinued during the time required for this examination.

A routine gallbladder study requires that the patient take nothing by mouth after his evening meal the day preceding the examination with the exception of the tablets containing the opaque medium. The evening meal the day prior to the examination is usually fat free with no cream, butter, or fried foods. The best results are obtained if for the evening meal the patient is on a low residue type of diet which includes fruit juices, dry toast, or food of a similar nature. Approximately 1 hour after the evening meal the patient is asked to take several tablets at 5-minute intervals. The tablets should be swallowed whole, not broken up or chewed. Breakfast is withheld the day of the examination and the patient reports to the x-ray department at 8 A.M., approximately 12 to 15 hours after his preliminary preparation.

Many radiologists believe it necessary for the patient to have two enemas; one to be given the night prior to the examination and one on the morning of the examination. If the patient is an outpatient, not under hospital care, it is necessary to give him very careful instruction as to the proper method to follow in preparing and taking an enema and at which times the enemas should be taken. In those instances when an enema is ordered in the morning also, the patient should understand that it be given at least a couple of hours prior to the examination. If this is not done, the possibility exists of the formation of gas in the bowel and this, in turn, could very well overlay the gallbladder area causing considerable difficulty in obtaining proper films.

This described patient preparation does not represent the opinion of all radiologists. There are many who believe that rather than a fat-free meal the evening prior to the examination, the patient should have a highly fatty meal. The basis for this theory is that the fat stimulates the gallbladder to empty itself of its *stored* bile and thereby is ready to receive the *dye-laden* bile. It must be remembered that if this method is to be used, the tablets should not be given immediately following the meal, but with a delay of 2 or 3 hours. Many authorities believe the patient should receive a dose of paregoric before taking the tablets to assist in alleviating nausea and purgation which sometimes follows the use of this kind of contrast medium.

Preliminary fluoroscopy and scout films. When the patient arrives at the x-ray department for the gallbladder examination, one of several methods may be used for taking the films. In large departments where a great number of gallbladder examinations are done each day, it is helpful to have the radiologist examine the gallbladder fluoroscopically, possibly taking spot films of the area and marking the location of the gallbladder in various projections to eliminate the necessity of scout films. Since the gallbladder does not visualize extremely well fluoroscopically, it is wise to arrange the scheduling in such a fashion that the gallbladder patients are brought into fluoroscopy after the radiologist has fluoroscoped some gastrointestinal patients. When this is done, the radiologist's eyes are well adapted and he will more readily make out the shadow of the gallbladder. When fluoroscopy is used, it eliminates the necessity for a scout film and aids the technician to the extent that the radiologist can tell more exactly what films will best demonstrate the gallbladder.

It must be remembered that the gallbladder is not in a fixed position in the abdomen and that its location will vary markedly from patient to patient. For example, in the obese patient the gallbladder is much more likely to be high than in the thin patient. If fluoroscopy is not used in locating the gallbladder or if, as is possible under some circumstances, fluoroscopy is used and the gallbladder is still not located, then it does become necessary to take a scout film of the gallbladder area (Figs. 7-3 and 7-4).

Patient explanation and care. Before beginning the examination, the technician should carefully go over the details of his preparation with the patient to make sure that the proper procedure has been followed and that the dye tablets have been taken as indicated. It is wise to find out whether the patient had any reaction from the dye, particularly whether any vomiting occurred and, if it did occur, at what time following the ingestion of the dye. When this type of opaque material is used, it is expected that there will be some catharsis, and if this has occurred to a marked extent, it may well affect the gallbladder shadow. This preliminary information, if it departs from normal, should be given to the radiologist before commencing the examination.

Inasmuch as the gallbladder is not in a fixed location, it is usually necessary to take several different projections of the area. If these projections are to be successful, it is necessary that the patient be informed thoroughly of what is to be expected of him to accomplish any of the positions. The technician should exercise all possible care in adjusting the body to make the patient as comfortable as the circumstances will permit. Usually the examination will start with

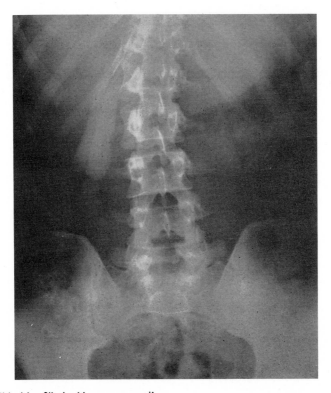

Fig. 7-3. Gallbladder filled with opaque medium.

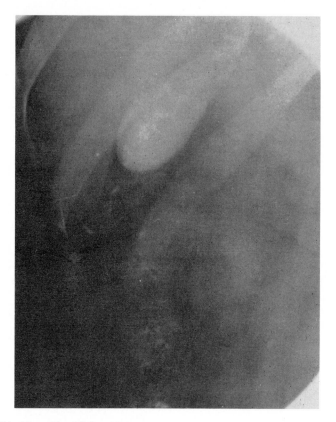

Fig. 7-4. Gallbladder with radiolucent stones.

the patient in the prone position. The technician should be certain that the patient's head is comfortable and that the arms are in a relaxed and comfortable position. The use of sponge padding or folded towels is indicated wherever there are bony protuberances. The ankles and feet should be supported in such a fashion that the weight of the feet is not on the toes.

If it is necessary to take a scout film for the purpose of locating the gallbladder within the area, this film should be taken with the patient in the prone position, using a 10 × 12 film. The technician should immediately process this film and show it to the radiologist to determine what further films must be taken. Normally these may include posteroanterior, oblique and lateral decubitus, and upright films, as well as an occasional anteroposterior, Trendelenburg's anteroposterior or Trendelenburg's posteroanterior film. Often these films are dependent upon one another to the extent that the following film is not taken unless an indication on the film which has just been taken previously dictates the additional position. It is, therefore, wise to inform the patient that this circumstance exists, that the doctor will have to see many of the films before deciding what his next film will be, and that the examination may be of considerable length. If the technician neglects to so inform him, the patient will often think that each of the films already taken was a failure or did not "turn out." He will have the idea that he is not in competent hands with a resultant lack of confidence which may well affect his opinion of the diagnosis when it is made by the radiologist.

In most instances the gallbladder films are made on the complete expiration phase of respiration since this is the phase in which the patient will be most relaxed. However at times, due to the location of the gallbladder, it may be necessary to take the film on inspiration in order to cause the gallbladder to shift to a lower point to become clear of obstructing gas. It is well, therefore, for the technician to practice respiration with the patient so that at the time of the film the right phase of respiration will be obtained.

After films satisfactorily demonstrating the gallbladder have been obtained, it is the usual practice to give the patient some type of fatty meal. This may be in the form of an eggnog or a glass of cream and milk or one of several commercial fatty meals available. It must be carefully explained to the patient that further films will be necessary following the fatty meal. If the patient is permitted to leave the department for this purpose, the exact time of his return must be thoroughly understood. Forty-five minutes to 1 hours after the ingestion of a fatty meal is sufficient lapse to take the after-fatty meal films. If the patient's gallbladder is functioning properly, the fatty meal will cause it to partially empty the dye-laden bile within the gallbladder and thereby demonstrate gall bladder function.

It is well for the technician to remember a combination of two prime factors in radiography of the gallbladder. First, the gallbladder is a moving area within the body, and therefore, a fast exposure time is necessary. Second, it is an area in which detail is of extreme importance. Therefore, the best combination of factors available to the technician with the equipment at command must be used for producing detail and eliminating motion.

Cholangiography

Operative cholangiography will be discussed fully in the chapter on operating room procedures.

Postoperative cholangiography. The postoperative cholangiogram, however, might well be considered briefly here. This procedure involves injecting a contrast material directly into a T tube which has been left in the biliary ducts following the surgical removal of the gallbladder and exploration of the biliary ducts. The purpose is to examine the biliary ducts. The examination is often done several weeks after surgery.

The patient preparation is similar to that for a regular gallbladder examination with the exception that no contrast medium is given prior to the examination. The patient's postoperative condition may determine modification of the regular procedure. The contrast medium is administered at the time of the examination by the radiologist.

Intravenous examination. The third type of cholangiogram, now in more common use, is the intravenous cholangiogram, using one of the commercially available contrast media designed for the purpose. The patient follows the preparation used for the gallbladder series with the exception that no tablets are taken. The patient reports to the x-ray department and upon being admitted is questioned about results of enemas and known allergies such as a history of hives, hay fever, or asthma. (Allergic persons are more sensitive to contrast media and must be observed very closely.) He is placed on the x-ray table in the antero-posterior position and the radiologist administers the opaque medium intravenously. Due to the rather toxic effect of the material, administration usually is preceded by a sensitivity test and the actual administration is prolonged over a 5- to 10-minute period for the injection of approximately 20 ml. of the material. In some instances, this may be injected with the usual intravenous needle and syringe, or it may be administered intravenously, first mixing the medium with 5% glucose and allowing it to enter the vein in the same manner as used for intravenous fluids. This method is advantageous because the dye is evenly administered over a 10-minute period which precludes the possibility of an uneven administration of the dye which might occur when using a syringe.

Following administration of the dye, during which time the patient is observed closely for sensitivity, the patient is put into an oblique position with the right side elevated about 10 degrees. Approximately 10 minutes later, a scout film of the area is made and a series of films follow at intervals covering a period of at least 1 hour. The usual result is the outline of the biliary ducts at some time during the course of these films. A regular gallbladder series of films may be taken about 1 hour after the administration of the dye if the patient has not had the gallbladder removed.

The primary considerations of the technician in this examination are the provisions of comfort for the patient through a prolonged examination, the necessary explanations to the patient, and observation for dye reactions; the technician must also make available beforehand the equipment for emergency care.

INTUBATION

On occasion it is necessary to pass a long intestinal tube through a patient's nose and into his stomach and small bowel when he has an obstruction in the small bowel, possibly due to a tumor. The swallowed air and the normal gastrointestinal secretions cannot pass beyond the obstruction, and therefore cause distension and great discomfort to the patient. Before the obstruction can be surgically removed or until the condition is alleviated medically, the patient's distension needs to be relieved by withdrawing these intestinal contents through suction and the subsequent decompression of the gastrointestinal tract (Fig. 7-5).

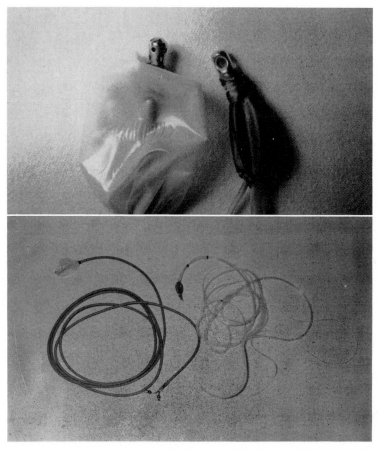

Fig. 7-5. Intubation. Two types of intestinal tubes, each with two lumens so that after it is swallowed and passed through the pyloric sphincter under fluoroscopy the balloon can be inflated with mercury or water, making its passage easier with peristalsis.

This situation was described in an earlier chapter and is referred to only because fluoroscopy is occasionally necessary. By actually viewing the tube fluoroscopically, its passage can sometimes be facilitated and it can be guided through the pyloric sphincter into the duodenum by mechanical means or by palpation of the area.

The patient is usually acutely ill when he is brought to the x-ray department to have this procedure done. Anything the technician can do to facilitate the passage of the tube, expedite the patient's stay in the department, or make his stay more comfortable is essential. The following suggestions are offered:

1. The attending physician usually brings the tube which should be in a basin of ice, making it stiff and easier to swallow.

2. Ask the patient to blow his nose to remove any obstructing mucus.

3. The tube should be well lubricated with KY jelly.

4. Provide a glass of water so that the patient can sip it while the tube is being swallowed.

5. The tube is passed more easily if the patient is sitting up.

Following intubation, the tube is usually attached to a suction system and the gastric contents removed before the leaded or mercury end of the tube is encouraged to pass on through the pyloric sphincter. After about one-half hour of frequent small advances of the tube, it is usually into the small bowel. It is checked under fluoroscopy, and the patient is returned to the station.

BRONCHOGRAPHY
Its definition and use

The bronchogram is a radiographic examination of the bronchi and their branches following the injection of iodized contrast material. The name "bronchial tree" is used to describe this area because the trachea branches out into two main bronchi, each in turn having several branches closely resembling the appearance of a tree.

Bronchography is helpful in determining the presence of foreign bodies. Children are frequently affected in this instance when they may have choked on a pin, coin, or other small object. Instead of swallowing it, spitting it out, or coughing it up, it may find its way down the trachea and lodge in one of the bronchi. A bronchogram then helps localize the foreign body before it is removed through a bronchoscope.

A more general use of the bronchogram is in the investigation of the extent and area of involvement of bronchiectasis, a condition in which the bronchi are dilated due to chronic suppuration. Probably the largest percentage of bronchograms are done for the purpose of diagnosing tumors of bronchogenic carcinoma.

Procedure and care of the patient

It is wise for the technician to have available and ready all the supplies that will be needed before the patient is brought to the x-ray department. This would include the sterile tray with catheters of various lengths and sizes, which are inserted down the patient's throat into the trachea. It would also include instruments or supplies necessary for applying local anesthesia to the patient's throat in order to pass the catheter and to depress the cough reflex. Cocaine derivatives are generally used. Several large syringes are included in the tray into which is poured the iodized opaque material, which is subsequently injected through the catheter into the bronchial tree. The vials of contrast media should be placed in warm water to ensure free flowing and be more comfortable for the patient when the opaque is injected.

The technical calculations for the type of patient should be computed before the patient is brought into the room. If the patient is a baby or child with a foreign body lodged in the bronchus or if the patient's age or degree of illness suggest difficulty in carrying out the procedure, additional trained personnel should be available.

After the technician has made the patient as comfortable as possible on the x-ray table, a brief explanation of the procedure should be made by either the doctor or the technician. The patient should be told that part of the examination will be done under fluoroscopy in a darkened room, followed by films made in various projections. It is important for the patient to realize that the success of the examination is dependent on his resisting a strong urge to cough after the introduction of the opaque material. The presence of the iodized solution will make it difficult for the patient to resist coughing. This is a natural reflex action in the presence of foreign material, which in this case is actually the contrast medium. However, if the patient is instructed to breath in a rapid, shallow fashion, or "pant," the impulse to cough is somewhat lessened.

The doctor begins the procedure by applying local topical anesthesia to the pharynx and larynx to ensure less painful introduction of the catheter. When local anesthesia has been accomplished, the doctor will begin the introduction of the catheter into the trachea, observing its progress under the fluoroscope. The catheter used will be somewhat opaque to the x-ray beam, permitting it to be observed fluoroscopically. The technician during this portion of the procedure should be encouraging and comforting the patient and assisting the doctor in any movement of the patient. When the catheter has been passed into the trachea and has arrived at the branching off point of the bronchus being examined, the doctor instructs the technician to attach to the end of the catheter a syringe containing the opaque material. This is usually Dionosil, a somewhat viscous liquid which cannot be drawn up into the syringe. It must be poured into the barrel of the syringe very carefully. The technician will then start injection of the material, being careful to follow the doctor's instructions as to the start and rate of injection as he observes the opaque material flowing into the bronchus. In order to fill the area it will be necessary to rotate the patient carefully into the oblique and lateral positions. This portion of the procedure is done in the darkened room, and it is therefore imperative that the technician have additional syringes and opaque material and the flashlight with the red bulb easily available if required.

Teamwork between the doctor, patient, and the technician is necessary for a successful bronchographic examination. During the fluoroscopic examination the doctor will be taking spot film radiographs of areas of interest. The tendency of the patient to cough complicates the examination as soon as the opaque material begins entering the bronchus. At this point the shallow, rapid breathing mentioned earlier is helpful, but it must be suspended, of course, during the making of the radiographs. When the bronchus or bronchi are filled, the lights are turned on and the technician positions the patient, making a series of radiographs in various patient positions. It is in this stage of the examination, when the bronchi are most filled with the foreign material of the contrast medium that the patient has the most difficulty controlling coughing. Unfortunately, it is also at this stage that such coughing must be prevented, since it spreads the opaque material into the lung fields, ruining the chance for a proper diagnosis of the films. Immediately on completion of the radiographs the technician should allow the patient to give way to the suppressed desire to cough, having available an emesis basin, towels, or paper tissues. Under no circumstances should he be given water to drink to help clear his coughing, since the throat is anesthetized. This may well cause the patient to aspirate or choke rather than swallow the water. For this reason all food and fluid is withheld from these patients for several hours following bronchography. Postural drainage is usually ordered by the patient's attending physician. In this treatment, the patient lies prone on his bed with his head and shoulders properly supported over the edge of the bed. This helps in draining out any opaque oil which remains in the bronchial tree.

Bronchography is not a complicated examination as far as the technical aspects are concerned. The films required are routine type of chest positions. The entire success therefore is dependent on constant patient care and reassurance during the procedure, careful teamwork, and fast accurate technique to complete the procedure for added patient comfort (Fig. 7-6).

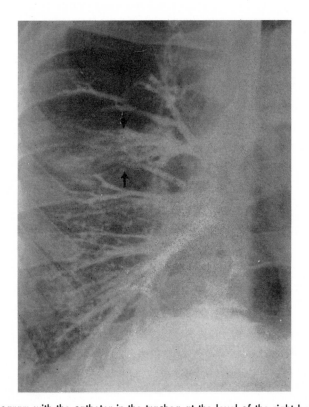

Fig. 7-6. Bronchogram with the catheter in the trachea at the level of the right bronchus.

INTRAVENOUS PYELOGRAPHY
Definition and use

Intravenous pyelography is the radiographic examination of the kidney, ureters, and bladder, with the contrast medium being injected intravenously. This is in contrast to retrograde urography which is the radiographic examination of the same area except that the contrast medium is injected directly into the ureters through cystoscopy. An intravenous pyelogram is generally the procedure of choice, since it is easier to do and requires no operative risk for the patient. Moreover, since the dye is injected intravenously and is circulated through the blood stream and then concentrated and excreted in the urinary tract, it is also a test for renal function. Cystoscopy and retrograde urography provide for direct injection of contrast media and a subsequent concentration of dye in the urinary tract at one definite, foreseeable time. This does provide good quality of contrast in films. However, intravenous pyelography is still the method of choice in examination of the kidney, ureter, and bladder unless cystoscopy was planned for the patient anyway or unless renal function is poor and the dye could not be concentrated to the extent where it would allow good visualization. Intravenous pyelography is helpful in diagnosing tumors, presence of stones, malformations, and other conditions.

Patient preparation

For a successful examination, the colon, which lies in front of the area to be viewed, needs to be as free as possible of feces and gas. This, together with dehydration of the patient, so that the dye is more concentrated at one given time, allows the film to be of greater diagnostic quality. The patient is usually given 2 ounces of castor oil or milk of magnesia between 4 and 6 P.M. the day prior to the examination. A light supper may be eaten but no food or liquid is allowed until the examination is completed the following day.

The request for an intravenous pyelogram by the referring physician or attending physician should include the usual diagnostic possibilities and a statement by him, too, as to whether or not there are any contraindications for the use of Pitressin. If the patient has a history of high blood pressure, heart disease, jaundice, or some other conditions, Pitressin is not administered. Pitressin is not used routinely in all examinations but is especially necessary where the patient has been poorly prepared physically. Acting as a smooth-muscle stimulant, it causes the patient to expel flatus and fecal material, and empty his bladder within a few minutes after it is administered. A previous section describes in detail the administration of Pitressin, its hazards, and technician responsibilities.

Procedure and care of the patient

Because there is some risk of a severe sensitivity to the contrast medium, the technician should have available for the radiologist the usual emergency equipment of stimulants, syringes and needles, tourniquet, blood pressure apparatus, and oxygen. Following the injection of a contrast medium, serious reactions occasionally occur. The patient who has such a reaction can be treated immediately if the x-ray room has been properly equipped with the necessary emergency treatment equipment. It is not uncommon for many patients to experience slight reactions such as increased respiration, increased perspiration, spasm, or pain in the blood vessel being injected.

The patient is placed on the x-ray table in a supine position. A preliminary or scout film is made and shown to the physician. If no objectionable gas shadows are present, the radiologist is called into the x-ray room to administer the opaque material. In most instances, he will either do a skin test or place a small drop of the material on the patient's conjunctival sac to observe any iodine sensitivity.

Since the early films of an intravenous pyelogram are primarily for the kidney area, it is wise to drape the gonadal area of the patient with lead rubber sheeting to prevent undue radiation hazard. This is particularly true in a patient

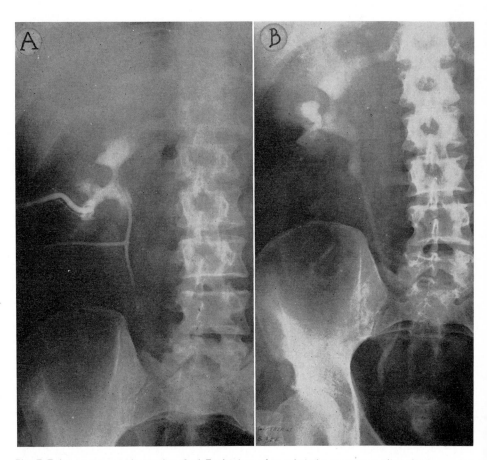

Fig. 7-7. Intravenous pyelography. **A,** A T tube is used to admit the opaque medium during a surgical procedure. **B,** Intravenous pyelogram after removal of compression.

under 30 years of age or in the case of a child or a pregnant woman. The doctor then selects a syringe and fills it with the opaque material and slowly makes the intravenous injection over a period of 3 to 5 minutes. In most instances shortly after the injection the technician takes the first radiograph.

A compression device frequently made of balsa wood or some other mechanical device is placed on and strapped across the patient's lower abdomen. Compression is thus applied on the ureters to keep the opaque material in the kidneys for a long enough period to obtain the necessary radiographs. Following a series of radiographs made at the requested time intervals, usually 10, 25, and 45 minutes after the injection, the compression is removed and a film is made of the ureters and bladder. Depending on the results of these, further films may be necessary or the examination may be terminated.

In recent years much use has been made of the drip intravenous pyelogram or the hypertensive intravenous pyelogram. These examinations basically differ from an ordinary intravenous pyelogram as described only in the manner in which the contrast medium is administered. In the drip intravenous pyelogram

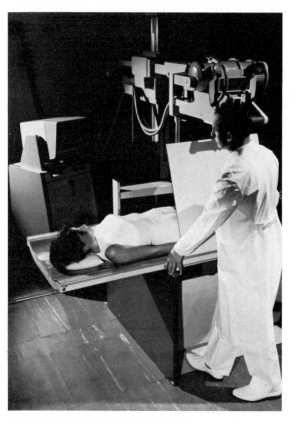

Fig. 7-8. Zonography may be done on this x-ray unit.

the contrast medium is mixed and administered, usually, from a bottle suspended on an intravenous stand. The purpose is to administer the contrast medium very slowly; this test is used where kidney function is poor.

It is extremely important that the patient understand the reason and necessity of compression. It is unusually uncomfortable for him, especially over a half-hour period or longer, and any kindness or word of understanding sympathy by the technician is greatly appreciated. The patient may feel, too, that the technician has forgotten him in the necessary time intervals between films. If he understands, however, that the procedure involves not one but a series of several x-rays at different times, the uncomfortable waiting on the hard x-ray table with compression on his lower abdomen will be better endured. Supplying any comfort device, pillow, or blanket that can be used while the patient is lying waiting for a subsequent picture shows thoughtful concern for the patient (Fig. 7-7).

The use of an examination called zonography is receiving wide acceptance, particularly in examinations involving the kidneys or the gallbladder. A zonograph is, in reality, a thick tomographic cut of the area under question and has the advantage of producing a radiograph which blurs out all structures and gases above and below the area of interest (Fig. 7-8).

The technician has several responsibilities in the intravenous pyelogram procedure which have nothing to do with x-ray technical skills. They are the following:

1. Making sure that the request for examination has on it all necessary information.

2. Having all necessary emergency supplies ready and available at the side of the x-ray table.

3. Never attempting the examination unless a physician is immediately available.

4. Maintaining a sense of responsibility in observing patient reaction during the procedure.

5. Making sure that no more compression than necessary is applied.

6. Properly explaining the procedure to the patient and understanding his discomfort.

REFERENCES

1. Braasch, W. F., and Emmett, J. L.: Clinical urography, Philadelphia, 1951, W. B. Saunders Co.
2. Brown, A. F.: Medical nursing, ed. 3, Philadelphia, 1957, W. B. Saunders Co., pp. 172-173.
3. Clark, B. G., Phillips, R. I., Goade, W. A., and Ettinger, A.: Recent advances in radiography of the urogenital organs, X-ray Technician **26:**175, 1955.
4. Cratens, J. E.: Physiology of the liver and gallbladder in relation to their radiographic study, X-ray Technician **15:**144-146, 157, 1944.
5. Deutschberger, O.: Fluoroscopy in diagnostic roentgenology, Philadelphia, 1955, W. B. Saunders Co., pp. 476-704.

6. Drum, H., and Fry, M.: Cholecystography, physiological and technical aspects, X-ray Technician **26**:261, 1955.
7. Dubois, E. C.: Hints on the management of a colostomy, Amer. J. Nurs. **55**:71, 1955.
8. Epstein, C. C.: Coronary insufficiency following intravenous pyelography, Calif. Med. **79**:406-408, 1953.
9. Hammer, L. G., Sawyer, J. G., Monica, Sister, and McKnight, J.: The three-maneuver enema, Amer. J. Nurs. **62**:7273, 1962.
10. Harper, F. R.: Pre- and post-operative care of patients for bronchoscopy, Hosp. Prog. **29**:378, 1948.
11. Harmer, B., and Henderson, V.: Textbook of the principles and practice of nursing, New York, 1955, The Macmillan Co., chap. 30.
12. Ingram, M. D., Jr.: Intravenous pyelography, X-ray Technician **24**:86, 1952.
13. Kerr, H. D., and Gilles, C. L.: The urinary tract: a handbook for diagnosis, Chicago, 1944, The Year Book Publishers.
14. Lesmeister, Sister V.: Cholangiography, X-ray Technician **25**:346, 1954.
15. McClain, M. E., and Gragg, S. H.: Scientific principles in nursing, ed. 5, St. Louis, 1966, The C. V. Mosby Co.
16. Merrill, V.: Atlas of roentgenographic positions, ed. 3, vol. 2, St. Louis, 1967, The C. V. Mosby Co.
17. Meschan, I.: Roentgen signs in clinical diagnosis, Philadelphia, 1956, W. B. Saunders Co., chaps. 25-30.
18. Montag, M. L., and Swenson, R. P. S.: Fundamentals in nursing care, ed. 3, Philadelphia, 1959, W. B. Saunders Co., chaps. 15, 16, 18, 21, 31.
19. Naterman, H. R., and Robins, J. A.: Cutaneous test with diodrast to predict allergic systemic reactions from diodrast given intravenously, J.A.M.A. **119**:491-493, 1942.
20. Rhinehart, D. A.: Roentgenographic technique, Philadelphia, 1954, Lea & Febiger, pp. 206-209, 357-359, 373-377, 385-403.
21. Rigler, L. G.: Outline of roentgen diagnosis, Atlas Edition, Philadelphia, 1938, J. B. Lippincott Co., Sections 6-9.
22. Sante, L. R.: Manual of roentgenological technique, ed. 12, Ann Arbor, Mich., 1945, Edwards Bros., Inc., pp. 198-214, 240-241, 248-251.
23. Scoggins, M. L. C.: Preparing patients for x-ray examination, Amer. J. Nurs. **57**:76, 1957.
24. Singer, A. G., Jr.: Comparison of intradermal and ocular methods of testing for sensitivity to Diodrast, Amer. J. Roentgen. **59**:727, 1948.
25. Starch, C. B.: Fundamentals of clinical fluoroscopy, New York, 1951, Grune & Stratton, Inc., chaps. 4-6.
26. Utz, D. C., and Thompson, G. J.: Evaluation of contrast media for excretory urography, Proc. Staff Meet. Mayo Clin. **33**:75-80, Feb. 19, 1958.
27. Wangensteen, O. H.: Intestinal obstructions, ed. 3, Springfield, Ill., 1955, Charles C Thomas, Publisher, chap. 6.

Chapter 8

Neuroradiography

The field of neuroradiography includes those examinations that are concerned with the brain and central nervous system. The pneumoencephalogram, the ventriculogram, the myelogram, and the cerebral and carotid angiogram are examples of this kind of procedure. Each may be used to assist in the diagnosis of neurologic conditions or as a diagnostic measure preceding neurosurgery. In each instance, a contrast medium is introduced; this may be an opaque contrast medium in some cases or a nonopaque contrast medium in other cases.

Pneumoencephalography is a procedure in which the ventricular and subarachnoid spaces are visualized radiographically by using air or gas as the contrast medium. The technique consists of withdrawing cerebral spinal fluid through a needle placed in the subarachnoid spaces in the spine and then injecting the air or gas. The air does not completely fill all parts of the ventricular and subarachnoid spaces at one time, so it is necessary to obtain radiographs in a variety of positions in order to delineate all parts of the ventricular system. Pathology or disease which can be diagnosed by the pneumoencephalographic procedure may also be evaluated by using an angiogram as the procedure. The condition of the patient can be a determining factor in the choice.

Ventriculography, a procedure which was commonly used in the past, has lost favor in recent years because of improved pneumoencephalographic and angiographic techniques. In the ventriculogram the examination is carried on in the operating room and involves two trephine holes through the skull over the occipital region of the head. Needles are then placed directly into the ventricles of the brain, and the ventricular fluid is withdrawn and replaced with air. This procedure does not change the intracranial dynamics or balance of cerebrospinal pressure to the extent that is true of pneumoencephalography. Hence, it was considered to be a safer procedure if the patient concerned had a space-occupying intracranial lesion. This procedure, of course, is technically more complicated because of the surgical implications involved.

Myelography is a roentgenographic study of the subarachnoid spaces of the spinal canal using a contrast medium. As is true in pneumoencephalography, a spinal needle is inserted into the subarachnoid spaces in the area below the questioned involvement. After spinal fluid is withdrawn through the needle, a contrast medium is injected, and its passage is observed and studied in the spinal canal, particularly at the point of obstruction. Myelography is helpful in the diagnosis of various types of spinal cord tumors, cysts, and ruptured intervertebral discs.

Angiography enables the visualization of the blood vessels of the head and neck and is performed by inserting a needle into the carotid artery or by using a catheter inserted into an artery, followed by the injection of a contrast medium. The placement of the catheter is usually under image-intensified fluoroscopic control. During and following the injection of the contrast medium, a rapid series of films is made as the contrast is quickly circulated in the circulatory pattern, enabling the radiologist to discern any displacement, obstructions, or abnormality of structures delineated.

PATIENT CARE AND TEAMWORK

Neuroradiographic patients are likely to be persons who are uncooperative because of medication or because of their neurologic conditions. The degree of cooperation will vary from patient to patient. The radiographic technician should anticipate poor cooperation and should be prepared to make the best possible use of equipment and accessories available to ensure immobilization and to establish a short exposure time technique.

In the case of the encephalogram, there is always time between each film to position the patient properly. The technician should not become hurried in these examinations because of the patient's condition. Speed is essential but not if it is going to result in a lack of good patient care and a poor film series which may require repeating the entire examination.

Because of the risk involved in these examinations, and particularly the risk due to repeat examinations in case of personnel failure, it is essential that the radiologic technologist, the radiologist, and personnel of other medical disciplines concerned with the examination operate as a team. For example, care should be taken to see that the neurosurgeon, if he is concerned in the examination, is well aware of the difficulties likely to be encountered by the technician in the performance of the technical functions of the procedure. The technician should have some basic understanding of the problems of the physician making the injection of air or other contrast media. The consequence of error involved in the procedure makes this teamwork essential.

PNEUMOENCEPHALOGRAPHY
General conditions

It is a common practice before a pneumoencephalogram is done for the patient to have a lumbar puncture or spinal tap, the purpose of which is to determine the pressure of the cerebrospinal fluid. An increased pressure is one indication that there may be a space-occupying lesion and would influence the neuroradiologist's approach to the examination. Depending upon the existing conditions an increased pressure might dictate that the pneumoencephalogram be abandoned as the diagnostic procedure or that a minimal air injection approach be used.

Although the area at the site of the spinal puncture is anesthetized, in many cases it is probable that the patient would have received some tranquilizing medication or sedation prior to the start of the examination. Normally a spinal tap is performed with the patient in the lateral recumbent position. However, for the pneumoencephalogram a lumbar puncture is done with the patient sitting upright if possible. The sitting position enables the air, which is lighter than the cerebrospinal fluid, to travel more easily to the intracranial spaces.

In the past, the spinal puncture and the injection of the air was often done at the patient's bedside in the ward. The patient was then transferred by litter to the x-ray department, where the necessary films were made. In recent years, as x-ray departments and radiologic technologists have become better equipped by training and with better facilities available, the entire procedure has been moved to the x-ray department. Eliminating the transportation of the patient from the ward to the department permits better control of the air and a better encephalogram result. The radiologic technologist, therefore, must now assume some of the duties of a scrub nurse when this examination is carried on in the x-ray department.

Careful preliminary planning is one of the keys to good patient care in all special procedure examinations. This is especially true in the neuroradiologic procedures. The successful pneumoencephalogram will involve a wide variety of radiographic accessories. The spinal tap and injection of contrast material requires the use of various pieces of sterile equipment. The need for immediate monitoring of the films or at least the preliminary films dictates some method of immediate and rapid processing. The possibility that the patient may faint or require resuscitation cannot be ignored. To have all supplies and accessories that might be required immediately available is mandatory. If the examination has to be interrupted because of lack of foresight in these preliminary preparations, poor patient care and a poor examination result.

Injection of contrast medium

When an encephalogram is to be done in the radiology department, including the injection of air, it involves the following: (1) The provision of a sterile tray with the following contents—drapes or towels, towel clips, and a variety of syringes and needles including spinal needles, a waste basin, medicine glasses, laboratory sample tubes, cotton balls, gauze sponges, and thumb sponges. (2) The provision of other supplies, such as sterile gloves for the physician, tincture of Zephiran or other disinfectant, Novocaine or other anesthetizing agent, and sterile transfer forceps. (3) A knowledge of the procedure by the technician and an understanding of sterile technique, as described in Chapter 4, are essential.

Review of reference points, lines, and planes

The technologist concerned in the technical processes of a pneumoencephalogram must be one who is very well grounded on skull positioning. It is proper to review these facts within the context of this description.

The reference points are as follows:

1. Intraorbital point, the lowest point on the margo infraorbitalis.
2. The supraorbital point, the highest point on margo supraorbitalis.
3. The external meatus.

The reference lines are as follows:

1. The infraorbital line is identical with the anthropologic base line (Frankfurter horizontal or Reid's base line) and is defined as a line between the infraorbital point and the upper boundary of the external meatus.
2. The supraorbital line passes through the supraorbital point and the upper boundary of the external meatus.
3. Orbitomeatal line extends from the external canthus of the eye through the external meatus.
4. The auricular line is perpendicular to the infraorbital line and passes through the external meatus.

The reference planes are as follows:

1. The median sagittal plane is the plane dividing the skull symmetrically into two halves.
2. The infraorbital plane is identical with the so-called anthropologic plane in which lies the anthropologic base lines (Reid's base lines).
3. The supraorbital plane, in which lie the supraorbital lines. This plane has, in several connections, replaced the orbitomeatal planes as a reference plane.

Examination technique

The illustrations in this chapter were chosen to demonstrate to the student technician some of the positions involved in pneumoencephalography and how they are accomplished when using sophisticated equipment. In this instance at the beginning of the examination, the patient is in the sitting position in an electrified rotating chair. Referring to Fig. 8-1, *B*, you will note that there is an aperture in the back of the chair; this is designed to permit the radiologist to have a convenient approach for the spinal tap.

The maneuverability of the chair permits turning the patient into any necessary positions; the air, therefore, can be carefully controlled and adapted to the capacity of the ventricular systems and that of the cisterns. The unit illustrated has linear tomographic capability, and this is found valuable, particularly in examinations of the basal cisterns.

The radiographs of the skull in the various positions in a complete pneumoencephalogram are not necessarily a standard series. Some radiologists will prefer one series of positions and others may prefer additional films in the series. The examination will begin usually, however, with the patient in the sitting position.

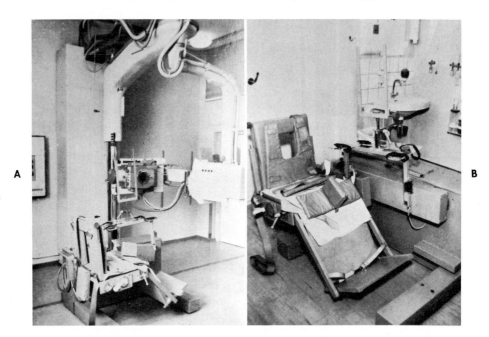

Fig. 8-1. A, Sophisticated apparatus used in the pneumoencephalogram examination. **B,** Close-up view of a tilting chair, which permits the various positions described.

Following the spinal tap and injection of a minimal amount of air, a lateral projection of the ventricular system with the patient's neck somewhat flexed is made. This original film will be followed by a frontal posteroanterior projection with the patient continued in the sitting position, and at this time additional lateral films are a possibility. The patient then will be placed in the prone position by rotating the chair, and films will be made both in the lateral and posteroanterior projections. The series will continue with further maneuvering of chair and skull so that the air will move into the various areas of interest within the skull. The examination will continue with films made with the patient in the supine position. Figs. 8-7 to 8-9 are illustrations of some of these basic positions.

If a circular chair of the type shown in Fig. 8-1, *B*, is used in connection with a pneumoencephalogram, great care must be practiced in immobilizing the patient. A constant check on the straps and buckles and their condition is the technician's responsibility.

Pneumoencephalography, of course, can be accomplished without the highly specialized equipment shown in the illustrations of this chapter. One might use an ordinary skull unit and a conventional chair or x-ray table. However, the principles involved would be similar. The same radiographs must be obtained, and the contrast medium (air) must be maneuvered in a fashion to cause correct filling. This, of course, is accomplished by maneuvering the patient and the

Text continued on p. 154.

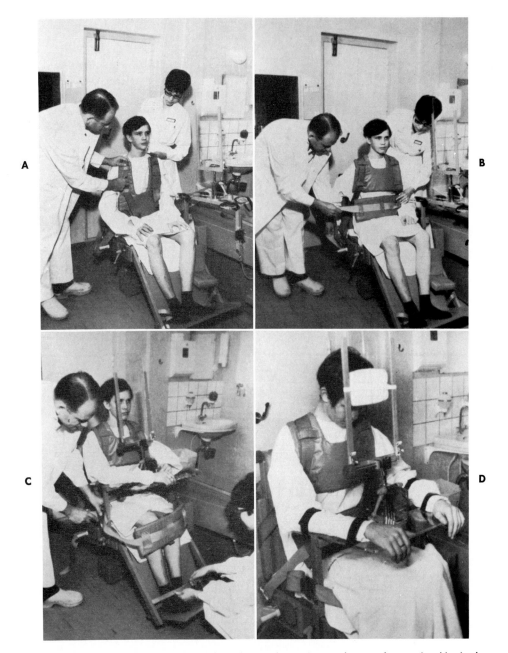

Fig. 8-2. Great care must be exercised in placing the patient and properly securing him in the tilt chair prior to the beginning of the examination.

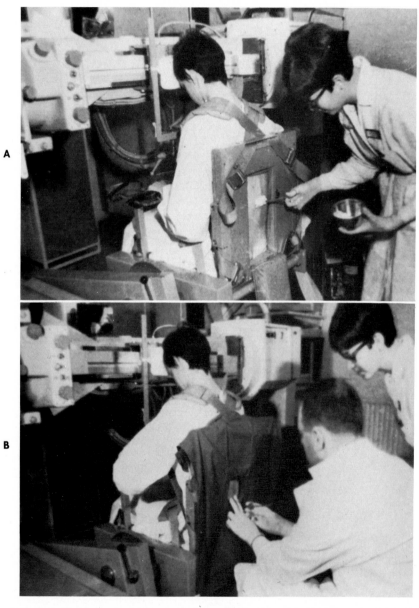

Fig. 8-3. A, Patient is prepared for a spinal tap. **B,** Injection of the contrast material (air).

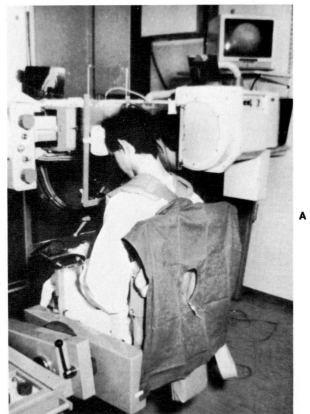

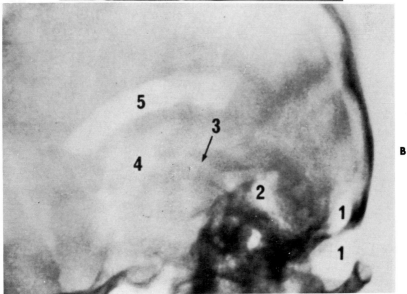

Fig. 8-4. Lateral projection of the ventricular system demonstrating: **1,** cisterna magna; **2,** fourth ventricle; **3,** aqueduct; **4,** third ventricle; **5,** lateral ventricle.

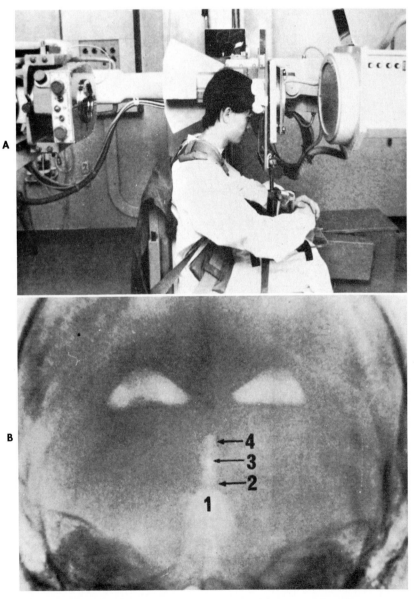

Fig. 8-5. Frontal posteroanterior projection of ventricular system demonstrating: **1,** posterior part of the fourth ventricle; **2,** anterior part of the fourth ventricle; **3,** aqueduct; **4,** third ventricle.

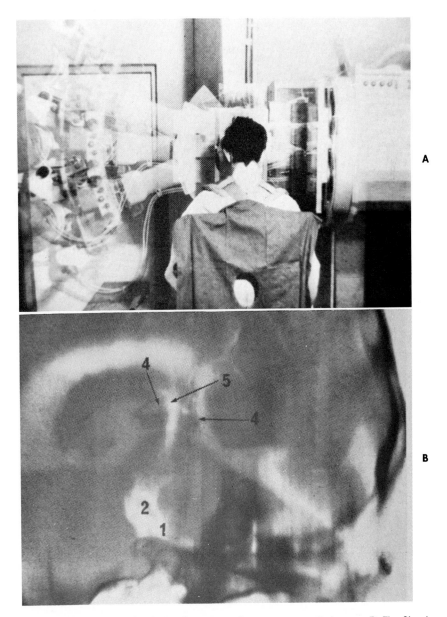

Fig. 8-6. A, Midline tomography during the course of a pneumoencephalogram. **B,** The film shows: **1,** the pontine cistern; **2,** the interpeduncular cistern; **3,** the quadrigeminal cistern; **4,** the wing of the ambient cistern.

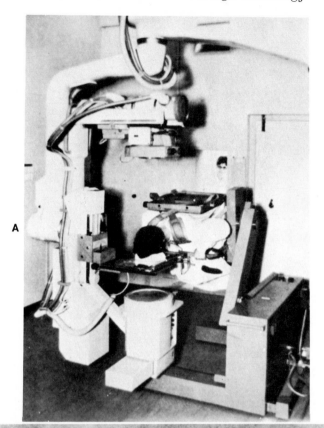

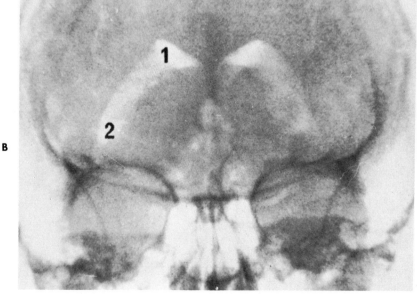

Fig. 8-7. A, Prone position, frontal posteroanterior projection. **B,** Demonstrated are: **1,** the body of the lateral ventricle; **2,** the posterior part of the temporal horn.

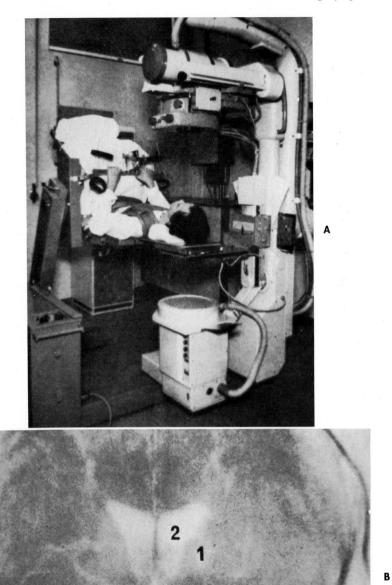

Fig. 8-8. A, Supine position for a frontal anteroposterior projection. B, Demonstrated are: **1,** the anterior horn; **2,** body of the lateral ventricle; **3,** the third ventricle.

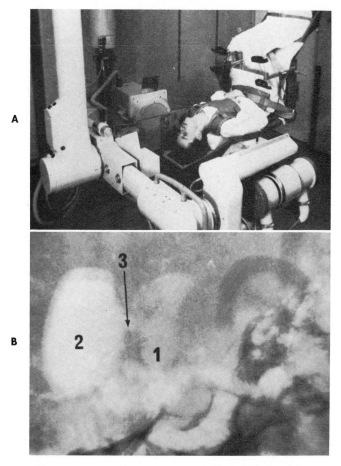

Fig. 8-9. Supine position with the hanging head to ensure filling of (1) the anterior recesses of the third ventricle, (2) the anterior horns, and (3) the foramen of Monro.

skull of the patient. Without specialized apparatus, the examination is more difficult to do and makes heavier demands on the patient and radiologist concerned with the examination.

Care of the patient during pneumoencephalography

Because the patient undergoing pneumoencephalography is usually under some sedation, he is generally rather groggy. Courteous behavior, simple explanations, and adequate privacy should not be discarded simply because the patient may be somewhat disoriented. A semiconscious patient should be treated with the same deference, care, and respect for comfort as all patients and with even greater concern for his safety.

Withdrawal of spinal fluid and the injection of air as a contrast medium is, in fact, the introduction of a foreign material. Sometimes this will produce shock

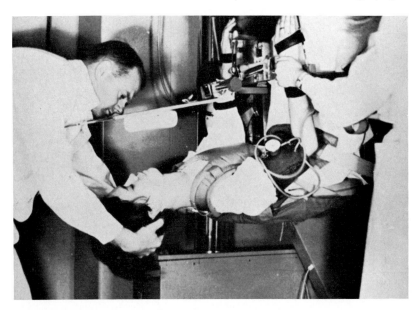

Fig. 8-10. Bringing the patient into a position by rotating the chair table backward. This position is used in case the patient faints during the course of the examination.

to the patient's nervous system. He may become pale, his pulse may become weak and thready, or he may feel faint or even actually faint. The technician must avoid becoming so immersed and involved in the mechanics of the procedure as to be unaware of the patient's condition and response.

The patient should never be left unattended upon completion of the examination. He may complain of headaches and nausea, and someone in attendance who will keep him lying down and quiet is indicated.

MYELOGRAPHY
Necessary radiographic equipment

Myelography, as do other procedures in neuroradiography, involves special equipment, specific patient care problems, and definite technician responsibilities. The x-ray table, if it is to be used to do all types of myelograms, including cervical, thoracic, and lumbar myelograms, should be constructed to motor drive to the vertical position from horizontal in either direction.

The table should be provided with a myelographic stop, a metal device which can be put into place to prevent the fluoroscopic assembly from descending toward the table beyond a certain point. The table should be equipped with shoulder braces to prevent the patient from sliding down when the table was tipped to a deep Trendelenburg position (see Fig. 8-11). The x-ray tube stand should be of a type that will permit being lowered sufficiently so that cross-table radiography during the examination is possible. The examination is more easily performed if the unit is one that includes an image intensifier with a

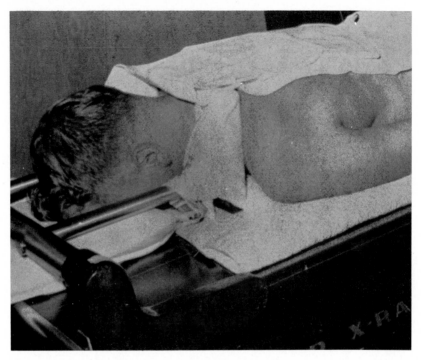

Fig. 8-11. Myelography. The patient is in position with his shoulders fitted well into the padded braces for a spinogram. The sterile drapes are already in place.

television camera and monitor so that all members of the team participating in the examination can be aware of the progress.

Responsibilities of the technician

The responsibilities of the radiologic technologist in assisting with a myelogram varies somewhat according to the methods preferred by the radiologist. All of the necessary preparations and equipment for the procedure should be ready and in a convenient location before bringing the patient into the x-ray room. The technician should have the necessary contrast medium and a myelographic tray ready on a table or instrument stand convenient to the x-ray table. It should include the usual spinal puncture type of apparatus. The technician should be sure that there are enough spot film cassettes on hand in a lead box conveniently near the x-ray table and should include any necessary grid cassettes for cross-table radiography. The patient's film folder with his recent spine films should be available for the radiologist to examine just prior to his starting his examination.

Procedure in positioning of the patient

Assuming that the x-ray room is equipped in the described fashion, the patient is brought in and placed on the table in posteroanterior position. His shoulders should be placed firmly against the padded shoulder braces, and every provision possible should be made for his comfort and safety. The radiologist, having scrubbed and put on the proper size gloves, will drape the patient's back before the spinal puncture. After anesthetizing the area, he will introduce the needle, usually in the lumbar area between the third and fourth vertebrae (lumbar vertebrae). Checking himself fluoroscopically, he slowly inserts the needle into the area, with many withdrawals of the stylette to establish whether the cerebrospinal fluid is being obtained. When he has punctured the dura, he then advances the needle slightly to make certain that the subarachnoid space is completely reached.

Ordinarily at this time he injects a minimal amount of the opaque medium and observes it fluoroscopically to make certain that the oil moves properly and, therefore, is in the space. When it is determined that the needle is in the proper position, a syringe with the contrast medium is attached to the hose, and the medium is injected. The amount will vary, depending upon the type of

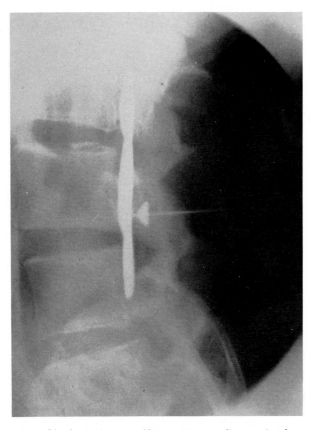

Fig. 8-12. Lateral view of lumbar spinogram. Note contrast medium coming from needle.

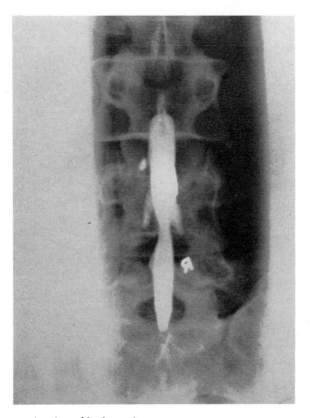

Fig. 8-13. Posteroanterior view of lumbar spinogram.

lesion being explored, although a minimal amount of 5 ml. is usually necessary, and often as much as 15 ml. is required.

After the contrast medium has been administered, the syringe is detached
and the needle is left in place in the spine. Because the radiologist must maintain sterile technique, it becomes necessary for the technician under the radiologist's direction to operate the equipment. The technician will motor drive the
table in the direction indicated by the radiologist, being extremely alert to follow his directions explicitly. The technician may be required to move the
fluoroscopic assembly to follow the contrast material as it progresses up the
spinal canal. The technician, in fact, becomes an extra set of hands for the radiologist during the course of a myelogram, a departure from the usual fluoroscopic responsibilities.

Prior to the maneuvering of the table and after the needle is in place, it is
essential that the technician check the myelographic stop to ensure that the
fluoroscopic assembly cannot come down to the patient's back and strike the
needle, which remains in place.

As the radiologist continues with the examination, an interruption of the flow

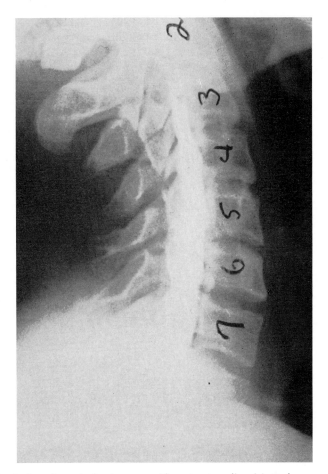

Fig. 8-14. Lateral view of cervical spinogram with contrast medium injected.

of contrast medium might indicate to him that he has reached the point of obstruction. At this time, spot films are usually taken, and it is necessary for the technician to make any equipment adjustments, place the cassettes in position, and operate the controls of the spot film device for the radiologist.

If the area under study is in the high thoracic or cervical region, the table may be tilted so that the feet are elevated slowly. Two technicians usually are required if the study is to involve the thoracic and cervical region.

One of the technicians will be at the head of the table, and as the dye begins to travel into the thoracic area, this technician will have to markedly extend the patient's head. The hyperextension of the head prevents the contrast medium from entering the cranial cavity. It is not possible to later recover the contrast medium through the needle in the spine if it has entered the cranial cavity.

Technologists assisting in myelographic examinations must be dependable, conscientious, well trained, and skilled in their duties and thoroughly aware of the hazards involved. The technologist should arrange his functions so that if the radiologist requires a cross-table lateral spine film during the course of the examination, the necessary grid cassette is available and a proper technique has been anticipated for the patient involved. It is possible and even probable that the cross-table film will be required at a time when the table is in the Trendelenburg position, and this complication should be anticipated. It is also necessary to provide a rapid method of processing films and returning them to the radiologist concerned with the myelogram. These films must be available during the course of the procedure and before the withdrawal of the contrast medium.

Upon completion of the examination, the radiologist will attach an empty syringe to the spinal needle in the patient's back and then direct the technologist to maneuver the table in a fashion to cause the contrast medium to puddle under the point of the needle so that it may be withdrawn.

The contrast medium used in these examinations is not of a type that is readily absorbable. If it is left in the spaces for any length of time, complications may ensue.

Disc puncture

A procedure closely related to the myelogram technically is called the disc puncture. It is usually done only in the lumbar area. This is a method by which a herniated intervetebral disc may be diagnosed by injecting contrast material directly into the disc. The technician's function in this examination is similar to the function carried out with the ordinary myelogram.

A principle difference in the procedure in a discogram is in the set up of the sterile tray. The tray usually includes a 20-gauge, 3½-inch spinal needle and also a 25-gauge, 5-inch needle. A 20-gauge needle is used to make the original spinal punctures of the disc. It is through the second needle that the opaque medium is injected. In the instance of the discogram, the opaque medium is not withdrawn following the examination.

Care of the patient

Now that the procedure of myelography has been described, several points of patient care become apparent. Most patients have a fear of spinal puncture and will be in need of reassurance. The injection site is always anesthetized locally and the patient suffers very little pain as a result of the injection.

However, tilting the patient to the point where he sometimes is nearly standing on his head can well cause fear and apprehension. Before the examination begins, the technician should carefully explain the positioning to the patient and show him the operation of the table. He should be shown the padded shoulder braces and restraint device and receive every possible assurance that he will be properly safeguarded during the procedure. If a cervical myelogram is being done, manipulation of the head should also be demonstrated before the actual procedure so that he understands the need for such an uncomfortable position and so that the technician and the radiologist may observe the patient's limitation of movement due to obstruction or pain.

NEUROANGIOGRAPHY

Development of new surgical technique and improvement of previously used surgical techniques usually parallel development of new or improved diagnostic radiologic techniques. This is true in the case of cerebral or carotid angiography. Cerebral angiography was first suggested and described by Moniz in 1927. At that time the contrast medium available was Thorotrast, which is a colloidal thorium dioxide. The disadvantages of using Thorotrast are that it can cause minor cerebral thrombosis and the development of chronic and strangulating granulomas of the neck whenever the contrast material leaks out of the artery into which it is injected percutaneously. Thorotrast also has a low-grade radioactivity with a half-life of 8 years. It did have the advantage of giving a sharper outline of the vessels but is considered more dangerous to the patient than contrast media in present use.

The development of better contrast media is a factor in the increased use of the angiogram in neuroradiology.

Cerebral angiography is indicated when surgical treatment is under consideration and when a precise diagnosis is required. Since there is some risk of reaction involved in even present-day contrast media, the examination is not done if differential distinction is of academic interest only. Contraindications to the angiogram include extreme age, advanced arteriosclerosis, severe hypertension, severe cardiac decompensation, and some other conditions.

There are several approaches to the angiogram used by the neuroradiologists. The examination is usually done under local anesthesia; however, it is possible that the patient would be under heavy sedation or even general anesthetic. In some instances the open method is used in which an incision is made and the artery is exposed for the insertion of the needle or a catheter. In other instances the percutaneous method may be used in which the needle is introduced through the skin and toward the artery. The x-ray equipment available in a department can dictate the approach that might be used in completing this kind of an examination.

Biplane cerebral angiography

A typical cerebral angiogram incorporating the use of the most modern equipment will be considered first. One of several available biplane rapid film units would be used in this instance. A biplane film unit permits the taking of several films rapidly, incorporating the use of two x-ray tubes, one of which exposes the lateral projection and one the anteroposterior projection. In this instance two x-ray generators are usually used, with each generator being responsible for the operation of one of the x-ray tubes. The advantages of this method are as follows:

1. Only one injection of the contrast medium is necessary to do the complete angiogram.

2. The contrast medium is in the same place at the same instance for the lateral projection and for the anteroposterior projection. The fact that the films can be taken simultaneously eliminates maneuvering the equipment and repositioning the patient's skull, which is required if the two projections are taken consecutively rather than simultaneously.

The disadvantages of biplane cerebral angiography are as follows:

1. Cost of equipment, since all of the angiographic devices available for biplane rapid film work are very expensive.

2. Controlling the cross-scatter of radiation which occurs when two tubes are fired simultaneously is a problem.

3. The positioning of the patient's skull in the simultaneous biplane angiogram results in the lateral projection having a radically increased part film distance with the usual loss of detail and magnification problems inherent with increased part film distance.

For these reasons the simultaneous biplane angiogram is not extensively used in neuroradiology.

The devices necessary for biplane cerebral angiography include two complete x-ray generators and controls, two tube stands, and two x-ray tubes. An alternative would be a specially constructed x-ray transformer and control which is capable of supplying half of its capacity to each of two tubes simultaneously. When the contrast medium is injected into the blood stream, it passes through the vessels of the brain through the arterial, capillary, and venous phases in a matter of 5 or 6 seconds under normal conditions. Several films in each of these stages are desirable. Therefore, the x-ray equipment is usually of high capacity, permitting rapid exposure time and an ability to recycle rapidly to permit the sequential exposures over the 5- or 6-second period.

Alternative methods

Most cerebral angiography is done using a single x-ray transformer and control in conjunction with a rapid film changer which can be positioned for either a lateral projection of the skull or an anteroposterior projection. Fig. 8-15, *B* and *C*, shows the examination being performed by this method. The patient's head is positioned on the film changer with the neck hyperextended to permit an easier approach in placing the needle in the vessel. This position complicates the technician's function in obtaining a satisfactory anteroposterior projection. It is necessary for the technician to use a rather exaggerated Towne's position with the angulation of the tube dictated in part by whether the patient has a short, thick neck or a long neck.

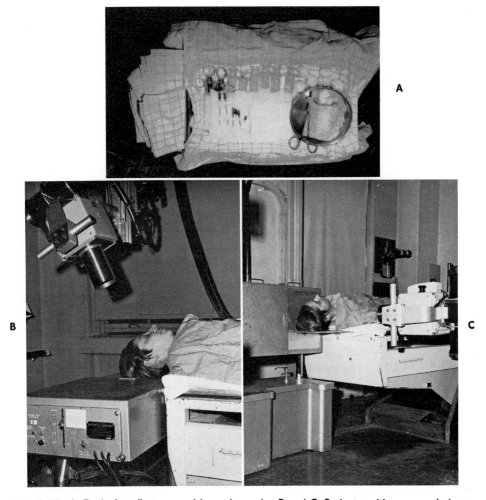

Fig. 8-15. A, Typical sterile tray used in angiography. **B** and **C,** Patient position commonly in use.

Assuming that the percutaneous approach is to be used, the examination would proceed in somewhat the following fashion:

1. The patient is placed on the x-ray table in the supine position with the skull supported on the film changer.

2. As the lateral projection is usually done first, the magazine of the film changer is positioned for the lateral projection (see Fig. 8-15, *B*).

3. The injection site is sponged using Zephiran or a similar disinfectant, and sterile drapes are positioned over the injection area.

4. The neuroradiologist inserts the needle at this point under sterile technique conditions.

5. When blood feeding back through the needle indicates to the neurora-

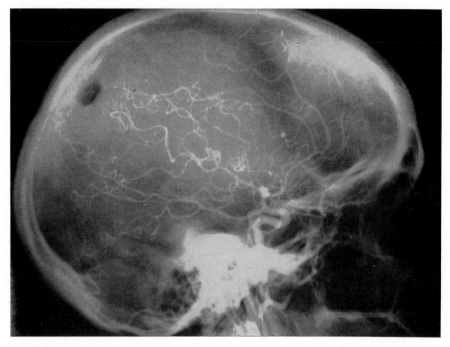

Fig. 8-16. Arterial stage in lateral cerebral angiogram.

diologist that he is in the artery, the syringe, containing the contrast medium is attached.

6. The injection is made by the neuroradiologist, and the technician activates the film changer to expose the films required in the lateral projection.

7. With the radiologist controlling the needle, the technician carefully lifts the patient's skull and rearranges the x-ray equipment and changer to prepare for the anteroposterior projection. Great care is necessary on the technician's part to ensure that the sterile field surrounding the injection site does not become contaminated and that no movement causes the needle to become disengaged in the blood vessel.

8. A second syringe containing contrast medium is now attached, and the neuroradiologist makes the second injection.

9. The technician activates the changer to obtain the films required in the anteroposterior position.

Care of the patient

The physician concerned in the examination usually assumes the responsibility of explaining the procedure to the patient beforehand. He will tell the patient the purpose of the procedure, the positions the patient will be required to assume, the sensations the patient may have as a result of the injection of the contrast medium, and similar information. Many of the patients will feel

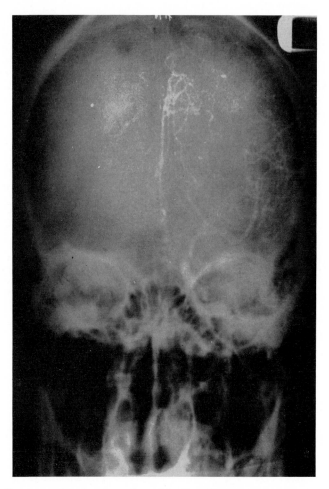

Fig. 8-17. Capillary stage in anteroposterior cerebral angiogram.

hot or flushed as the time of the injection of the contrast medium, some may have a choking sensation, and many will find the injection somewhat painful. If the patient knows what to expect, however, he will be more relaxed and can cooperate more fully.

It is the technician's responsibility to provide for the comfort of the patient by making sure that there is padding available under the bony protuberances and that he is covered, with privacy ensured at least to the degree permitted by the examination. The technician must have in mind all of the accessories and equipment that will be used during this examination and have them prepared and ready for use. As the injection of the contrast medium involves sterile technique, all necessary supplies and equipment conveniently available for use during the course of the examination is an additional responsibility of the technician.

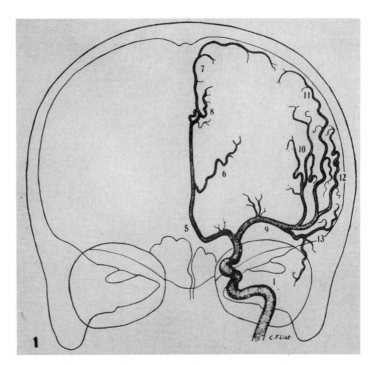

Fig. 8-18. Diagram outlining normal anteroposterior view of the cerebral artery system.

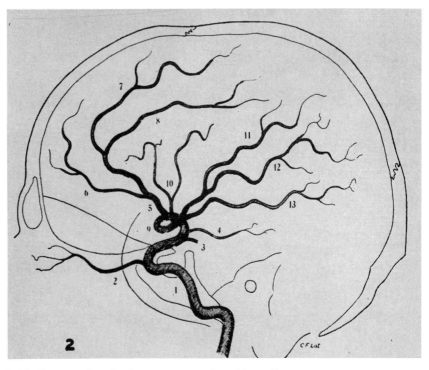

Fig. 8-19. Diagram of cerebral artery pattern viewed laterally.

The patient must never be left unattended following the examination until he is discharged to the care of the nursing staff in the ward. Occasionally a patient has an adverse reaction during the course of the examination, and therefore emergency kits, oxygen, and suction should be immediately available at the examination site.

There are many methods of approaching this kind of a procedure, some more sophisticated than the one described and some less sophisticated. The patient-care problem is common to all or any of the methods.

STEREOTAXIC TECHNIQUES IN NEURORADIOLOGY

Stereotaxy could properly be placed in the chapter on operating room radiography because this procedure is usually carried on in the operating room. It, however, requires a combination of techniques that involve neurosurgery and neuroradiography and further requires considerable specialized instrumentation. Stereotaxic operations were devised to permit a minimal surgical rather than a radical surgical approach to treatment of a certain condition. They are most commonly used for the surgical treatment of pain or for the treatment of Parkinson's disease.

The problem presented to a neurosurgeon in a stereotaxic operation is the introduction of a needle or an electrode to an exact point in the brain. This point could be an area where electrocoagulation could interrupt the function of pain-conducting fibers and therefore alleviate intractable pain in the head and neck from which the patient might be suffering. The point could also be at the location of the ansa lenticularis and globus pallidus in which case the aim would be to desiccate these areas which are responsible for the paralysis agitans (shaking) prominent in patients suffering from Parkinson's disease.

Because the patient's reaction must be observed during the course of the introduction of the needle or electrode, the operation is carried on with no anesthesia except for some local anesthesia at the site of the injection.

Radiography in stereotaxy is used basically to guide the surgeon who is introducing the needle or electrode into the brain. There are several different apparatuses used as the needle or electrode guide, but basically they resolve themselves into a head-holding device which is applied to the patient and fastened securely to his skull, in some instances, surgically. The function of this device is to hold the electrode or needle that is to be inserted in a very rigid position so that no uncontrolled deviation of the electrode can occur while it is being inserted. The patient is in a sitting position in an operating chair table. The radiographic problem that occurs is that a series of duplicate radiographs in two projections will have to be made during the course of the operation. These radiographs must be made under identical conditions as to position of tube, patient, and film. As the target in the brain is an extremely small area (plus or minus 1 ml.) distortion in the radiograph presents considerable problem.

In the highly sophisticated neurosurgery centers of the world, this problem is solved by having special x-ray apparatus with tubes mounted at a focal-film distance of 13 feet or more. This, of course, requires a special operating room with a tremendously high ceiling and also an operating room of good size to permit a 13-foot distance for the lateral projection. Thirteen feet is chosen as a focal-film distance in this instance because at this point no distortion in the radiograph or the parts being radiographed will occur.

Institutions that do not have these specialized rooms for the procedure will use x-ray equipment in fixed positions and a calculated distortion factor is computed and applied to the measurements to be made on the radiograph as to the location of the point of the needle or electrode.

In the instance of stereotaxic operations, the patient-care problem is, for the most part, handled by the doctors and the operating room nurses. The technician's contribution is to provide films of extreme accuracy and to be able to provide these repetitively without variations in technique or position. As a practicing member of the surgical team, the technician will have to be well grounded in sterile procedures and operating room techniques.

Chapter 9

Vascular radiography and fluoroscopy

GENERAL DEFINITION

In vascular radiography a contrast medium is introduced into the vascular system, making the arteries and veins stand out on a radiograph taken during or after the injection. Included in the general category of vascular examinations is the heart catheterization, which is the introduction of a catheter under fluoroscopic control into the blood vessels or into the chambers of the heart. Cerebral angiography, properly, is a vascular radiographic examination. In this book, however, the cerebral angiogram is discussed in the preceding chapter with other neuroradiologic procedures. The following examinations are classified as being vascular radiographic or fluoroscopic procedures:

1. Heart catheterization
2. Angiocardiography
3. Coronary arteriography
4. Peripheral arteriovenography
5. Abdominal aortography
6. Aortoarteriography
7. Carotid arteriography
8. Splenoportography
9. Renal arteriography
10. Pulmonary angiography
11. Installation of pacemaker
12. Rashkind's technique
13. Various types of venography
14. Various other arterial or venous injection procedures

HISTORY

Probably the beginning of heart catheterization under fluoroscopic control and of angiocardiography can be attributed to a German, Forssmann, who in 1929 passed a ureteral catheter through the veins of his right arm and into the right atrium of his heart. He attempted the injection of an opaque compound through this catheter but was unsuccessful in producing films of a diagnostic quality due to technical difficulties—not due to an inability to opacify the area. The first successful demonstration of opacified pulmonary vessels is generally credited to Moniz, de Carvalho, and Lima in 1931. These investigators used

Forssmann's technique of placing a catheter into the right atrium and injecting the opaque material into the veins of the elbow. They obtained a series of films showing the superior vena cava, the right atrium, the pulmonary arteries, the inferior vena cava, and the hepatic veins. The opaque material used was a sodium iodide solution. Reactions of a serious nature resulted in the abandonment of the examination for some years. Robb and Steinberg in 1936 and 1937 conducted a series of examinations using Diodrast as the contrast medium and reported minimal reactions to the material in a series of 215 injections in 123 persons.

At this point, impetus was generated by using heart catheterization and angiocardiography as diagnostic procedures, with radiologists, technicians, and manufacturers of x-ray equipment directing their efforts toward developing equipment and techniques that would permit extremely fast exposure times. They also developed a process of advancing films into the exposure area and removing them rapidly after exposure, the purpose being to have a series of radiographs of good quality with exposure times fast enough to minimize the loss of detail inherent in a moving liquid material, the opacified blood.

Other vascular radiographic procedures have followed a somewhat parallel course in development. For the past 15 or 20 years, vascular radiography and fluoroscopy has been the most dynamically changing field in the speciality of radiology. In a previous chapter of this book, the leading causes of death in the United States in 1900 were compared with those in 1948. In 1900, diseases of the heart and circulatory system were listed as one of the fourth or fifth causes of death. By 1948 heart and circulatory diseases had climbed into first place. Medical discoveries and investigations had relegated the previous leading cause of death to a minor role.

As circulatory disorders and heart disease became the number one killer, they also became the number one object of medical research. The intense effort put into this phase of medicine has resulted in the development of surgical techniques and diagnostic procedures and the introduction of new methods of treatment. As is true in any great advance in medicine, the development of new equipment and new skills was of paramount importance.

EVOLUTION OF X-RAY EQUIPMENT USED IN VASCULAR RADIOGRAPHIC AND FLUOROSCOPIC PROCEDURES

In general, the principal problem in vascular radiography is to discover methods of making a series of films of good contrast, density, and detail with extremely fast exposure times. It must be remembered that the x-ray technician is dealing with a rapidly flowing body of blood. The problem might be considered parallel to that of taking a series of still photographs rapidly following the dumping of a dye into the rapids of a river. Before the dye became diluted as the result of its mixture with water, films in every phase of its movement over a prescribed course would have to be taken very rapidly.

Because of the limitations of x-ray equipment, the early investigators in the various vascular radiographic examinations were forced to satisfy themselves with one or two films taken over a period of several seconds. The equipment limits dictated that these films would be made with comparatively slow exposure times. Catheterization of the heart under fluoroscopic control was difficult because the examination had to be performed in the dark. As the diagnosticians and their associates worked in developing equipment and techniques to permit better diagnosis of vascular abnormalities, the surgeons and their associates were developing surgical techniques and equipment to permit the correction of the abnormalities.

X-RAY EQUIPMENT IN THE
MODERN CARDIOVASCULAR SUITE

To solve the technical problems existing in the vascular radiographic and fluoroscopic area of radiology, it was necessary to make a multifacet attack on equipment design.

X-ray tubes

X-ray tubes have been developed with greatly increased heat storage capacity. These tubes permit many exposures to be made in sequence in an extremely short period of time. The modern x-ray tube will also permit each of these series of exposures to be of high energy. These two qualities have been accomplished without unduly increasing the size of the focal spot of the x-ray tube. Later in this chapter, in the discussions of individual examinations, the importance of this breakthrough is pointed out.

A recent development in x-ray tube manufacture that is very useful in many of the vascular radiographic procedures is the so-called magnification x-ray tube. The magnification x-ray tube is different from the average tube in that it has a decreased angle of the focal spot. This angle is usually in the nature of 10° rather than the conventional 15° to 17°. By decreasing the angle of the focal spot, it is possible to have a much smaller effective focal spot without sacrificing a high percentage of the ability to load this focal spot. This permits moving the film away from the patient and bringing the x-ray tube close to the patient with the resulting radiograph magnifying the details that will be resolved on the film. The ability to load this focal spot as the result of its new design permits radiography with comparatively little sacrifice in exposure speed. The technique is helpful in studying small vessels.

Exposure timer

The exposure timer of an x-ray unit has an important contribution to make toward the success of these special procedures. The ability to time x-ray exposures at the rate of 1/60 of a second or slower has been available to the profession for many years. In the instance of the equipment necessary for vascular radiographic examinations, however, a faster exposure time than 1/60 of a second is preferable. Also of great importance in the timing circuit is the ability of the x-ray timer to prepare for a rapid series of timed exposures. This ability is described as being the recycling time. Recycling means the elapsed time from the end of one exposure until the timer and x-ray unit are ready to make the following exposure. Older x-ray units were designed in a fashion that permitted this recycling to occur approximately once per second. In vascular radiography the possibility of making six to twelve exposures in 1 second is necessary. The design of x-ray exposure timers, therefore, has moved toward an extremely fast recycling time plus an ability to time an individual exposure in the millisecond range. Ideally, in most vascular procedures the time for exposure should be as fast as possible. Returning to our analogy of the dye in the rapids of a river, a person can visualize the dynamic movement that has taken place and the rate of exposure that would be necessary to catch every phase of such motion. The modern x-ray units in use in vascular radiographic procedures have the ability to time an individual exposure as fast at 1/360 of a second. An exposure time of this nature will stop motion almost completely.

X-RAY GENERATOR DESIGN

The x-ray generators (controls and transformers) used in these rapid film procedures have also been extensively revolutionized in the past years. The trend has been toward higher capacities with dependable stabilized control of milliamperage and kilovoltage. The auxiliary apparatus, which must be operated with these generators and must receive their power from them, necessitated a more complex control unit. Circuitry for the operation of many auxiliary devices had to be incorporated in the x-ray control. To minimize radiation hazards to patients and also to personnel, a need for high kilovoltage techniques became apparent. Many of the procedures require the simultaneous firing of two x-ray tubes, either from one generator or from a pair of generators. Inherently there is a calculated risk to the patient in undergoing vascular radiographic and fluoroscopic examinations. However, the modern x-ray equipment used during the procedures has minimized the chance for some of the failures experienced by the earlier investigators.

Image amplifiers and television circuits

Vascular radiography and fluoroscopy usually involves some surgical techniques. To carry these techniques out in a darkened room is a handicap. Many of the examinations require the introduction of a catheter into either the heart or some portion of the circulatory system. The catheter must be guided under fluoroscopic control. The location of the end of the catheter inside the human body must be well defined anatomically at all times.

The development of the image intensifier, with its companion developments of the possibility of cineradiography or televised fluoroscopy, has greatly simplified the technical approach to the many vascular procedures. The fluoroscopist using an image intensifier does not view the fluoroscopy screen, but rather by television monitoring or in some instances a mirror viewing system, he sees the image from the fluoroscopic screen multiplied many thousands of times in brilliance.

Image intensifiers, since their development, have improved in efficiency to the point that it is not uncommon for the image presented to be several thousand times greater in brilliance than that seen on the routine fluoroscopic screen. The brilliant image allows the fluoroscopist and other members of the team the use of their cone vision as they observe the image.

Cone vision permits better resolution of the details available in the observer's eye.

All vascular fluoroscopic and radiographic procedures are team efforts. The advantage of each member of the team being able to know what is going on fluoroscopically is apparent.

An additional advantage is that a patient is less apprehensive than he would be if he were being examined in a darkened room. Finally, the whole procedure carried on under televised fluoroscopy has an additional benefit in that the patient receives a reduced radiation dose than was formerly true.

Early in the development of these techniques, it occurred to many persons that a method of photographing the fluoroscopic screen with a movie camera would be of much help. This was technically possible in the early development of angiocardiography when the fluoroscopy was carried out under conventional fluoroscopic conditions. However, the exposure factors necessary were dangerous to the patient. In order to cause a conventional fluoroscopic screen to emit sufficient light to produce satisfactory movies, it was necessary to use extremely high milliamperage and kilovoltage, resulting in a heavy radiation dose to the patient. With the advantage of the image intensifier and its companion developments, the televised fluoroscopy equipment, cineradiography, and taped television recording of the image have become common. These two methods are probably best to study the dynamics of the flow of the opacified blood.

However, it is best that a cardiovascular suite be equipped with equipment to do biplane radiography as well as cineradiography. The advantage of cineradiography, aside from its obvious one of a study of motion, is that it can be more easily implemented during the course of the catheterization. If the patient's condition is critical or if the location of the catheter is at a critical point, a cine strip or a taped strip can be easily made. The biplane angiogram, however, with routine films taken in rapid sequence in two planes, has the advantage of better detail and the production of more informative type of film. The maneuvering of the equipment to position, placing the patient in proper relationship to the equipment, is more time-consuming in the biplane radiographic examination than in the cineradiographic examination. The biplane radiographic examination does, however, permit pinpointing abnormalities in two projections at the same instant. Experimental development of biplane-cine apparatus is well along, and many academic institutions have the capability of making such movies.

Another recent development in connection with cineradiography has been the development of circuitry which permits remoting a patient's electrocardiogram from the monitoring equipment on to a corner of a cine strip which is being made of the fluoroscopic image, and this can occur simultaneously. When studying the cineradiography following an examination using this technique, the electrocardiographic information that is present on the monitoring equipment is also present on the corner of the film and thus produces these two pieces of information for simultaneous viewing by the radiologist.

Rapid film changers

Originally all vascular radiographic procedures were studies using the one-film method. The physician would inject a contrast medium into the circulatory system of the patient and, by exposing one film after injection, gain some necessary information. However, it was apparent that many additional films in a short period of time would give better information. It was further determined that in many circumstances it would be helpful in arriving at a diagnosis if these films could be made simultaneously in two planes.

An attempt to get a series of films by rapidly transporting cassettes was the first approach to answering the problem. It was simple to construct a cassette changing device that would permit the taking of serial films at the rate of approximately one per second. Further study revealed that during the 1 second necessary to put a new cassette in the field with this kind of device, the contrast-laden blood could pass through a cycle which, if radiographed, would produce important information.

Various approaches were attempted to speed up film transport time and to develop faster recycling times and exposure times. One approach was the use of a roll film device. The basic mechanism of the original roll film device was adapted from an aerial camera used during World War II by reconnaissance planes. The camera had the ability to advance photographic film of large size at a rate of two frames per second. The unit was manufactured by the Fairchild Instrument Corporation. This corporation, in conjunction with several investigators, modified the serial photographic camera by installing a pair of intensifying screens (similar to those used in cassettes) in the exposure area. There is little doubt that this instrument contributed markedly to the beginnings of successful angiocardiography. Diagnoses, however, were still being missed because the rate of film advance was not rapid enough. Rigler and Watson, in conjunction with the Pako Corporation, developed a rapid film unit in which the film from a roll was advanced through intensifying screens. Following exposure, the exposed portion was automatically cut off and stored in a radiation-proof receiver. The unit permitted film advance at the rate of five frames per second and was a step in the proper direction. The unit was never developed for biplane radiography, which is necessary in many procedures. Two additional film-advancing units were developed in Sweden, and these units are the most widely used at the present time. In one of these changers, cut film is advanced into a pair of intensifying screens, where it is exposed and advanced into a receiver, the speed of film advance being, at its maximum, six frames per second. In addition, a roll film device of similar nature was developed which would permit the advancing of film at the rate of twelve frames per second at its maximum speed. The development of the x-ray units that would permit exposures repeated at the rate of twelve times per second, and the development of these two rapid film-changing units have been extremely helpful in the field of vascular radiography.

Heart catheterization table

The conventional radiographic-fluoroscopic x-ray table was not ideally suited for cardiovascular radiography and fluoroscopy. In routine heart catheterization, heart catheterization with selective angiocardiography, and many of the other vascular radiographic examinations in which a catheter is introduced, great care must be exercised in moving the patient. Disturbance of the location of the catheter point can result in outlining the wrong area during the injection of the contrast medium, and in certain critical areas the catheter point could start fibrillation. With these facts in mind, a table was designed with a sliding table top which permits movement of the table top with the patient lying on it without moving the patient. The course of the catheter can be observed fluoroscopically by slight movements of the table top in relationship to the image intensifier. If an angiocardiogram or other procedure is decided upon, the table top can be moved over the biplane changer, again without disturbing or moving the patient.

Another improvement has been the development of a greater focal-table top distance. The fluoroscopic tube under heart catheterization tables is 22 to 24 inches from the table top. This increased distance permits better detail on cineradiographic studies as well as better detail of the fluoroscopic image.

Ancillary equipment in the vascular suite

In addition to the complicated x-ray equipment that has evolved for the purposes of vascular fluoroscopy and radiography, much nonradiographic equipment is used. The use of anesthesia and contrast media, the introduction of catheters, and, in some cases, the condition of the patient require that the examination rooms be equipped for any type of emergency.

Occasionally, fibrillation will occur during an examination. Fibrillation causes disruption of heartbeat. An electronic machine called a defibrillator is used to bring fibrillation under control and restore normal heartbeat. At times, other complications may occur during an examination. The patient may have an allergic reaction to the contrast agent. Occasionally the patient may go into cardiac arrest. The well-equipped cardiovascular suite, therefore, must have emergency kits containing proper equipment and drugs. Suction apparatus and oxygen equipment must be available at all times.

In heart catheterization particularly and in other vascular procedures a multi-channel monitoring instrument is used. This instrument permits the recording of an electrocardiogram during the course of the examination. A second channel may be recording an electroencephalogram (electrical reaction in the brain). Other channels may be used to record pressures through the catheter as it is advanced into the various chambers of the heart. An instrument, called a transducer, is necessary for recording the pressures. It is attached by a stopcock to the end of the catheter outside of the patient's body. It converts the pressures it takes from the catheter into electrical signals, which are then fed into the monitoring system. All of these records are visualized on the multichannel unit while the catheterization is in progress.

Many laboratory instruments are used in cardiovascular radiographic suites. During the course of heart catheterization, blood samples are taken at intervals through the catheter. The samples are analyzed during the examination.

Sterile Instruments and supplies

The special procedures outlined in this chapter have one thing in common. They all involve surgical techniques to a degree. This means that the cardiovascular suite is, in reality, a minor surgery operating room as well as an x-ray examining room. Each of the vascular radiographic and fluoroscopic procedures requires the use of sterile packs containing the instruments and supplies necessary for the procedure. Typical sterile supply packs for cardiac catheterization contain the following, although individual preference by the physicians finally dictates the contents of the packs.

1. Catheterization pack
   a. Several mosquito forceps, both straight and curved.
   b. Allis forceps
   c. Tissue forceps
   d. Probe
   e. Needle holder
   f. Bard-Parker knife with blades
   g. Dressing and operating scissors
   h. Variety of syringes and needles
   i. Several small cruved cutting needles for suturing
   j. Suture material
   k. Three-way stopcocks and rubber tubing connections
   l. Several medicine glasses
   m. Sponges and stainless steel pans
2. Drape pack
   a. Two large drapes
   b. Four towels
   c. One large pillowcase and one small pillowcase
3. Arterial pack
   a. Several towels

    b. Some 5 ml. syringes
    c. A variety of needles from 22 to 25 gauge and medicine glasses
  4. Miscellaneous sterile supply
    a. Heart catheters
    b. Drip solution
    c. Sterilizing agents
    d. Sterile rubber gloves of various sizes
    e. Operating gowns
    f. Masks and caps

Early investigators discovered that one of the problems associated with vascular radiography was the rapid rate at which the contrast agent became diluted. Hand injection of the contrast material with a conventional syringe did not permit a large bolus (mass of liquid) to be released instantly into the blood stream. The time it took to push the plunger and empty the syringe was too long. Upon reaching the critical area to be filmed, the medium was too dilute to permit good contrast on the radiographs. The length of injection time permitted the heart to pump the contrast-laden blood over a longer period before filming was complete. The problem has been overcome by the development of power injectors. The plunger of the syringe on these units is propelled by gas under pressure. A large bolus can now be injected more rapidly than was possible with a hand-operated syringe. The shorter injection time results in less dilution of the contrast agent.

EVOLUTION OF THE CARDIOVASCULAR SUITE

Teaching hospitals and very large general hospitals have experienced a constant increase in demand for vascular radiographic and fluoroscopic diagnostic facilities. Whereas many of the examinations in this category require varying approaches, the group as a whole require the use of similar x-ray equipment and ancillary facilities. Ideally, this suite of rooms should include a large examination room, a smaller room for laboratory procedures, and a small storage-medical preparation type of area.

A common mistake is to make the general examination room too small. From the description of the equipment used, it is apparent that permanent installations occupy much floor space. The operation of the complicated equipment necessary to successfully carry on the examinations makes a large control booth area mandatory. The main examination room should have approximately 500 to 700 square feet of space, and the control booth, approximately 80 square feet. The laboratory connected to the main examination room, used for the medical technology procedures, should have approximately 120 square feet. The minor examination or minor surgery preparation room should also contain 120 square feet.

The design of a cardiovascular suite requires more than general architectural and administrative knowledge. The equipment in a standard examining room of this type requires auxiliary wiring circuits in the ceiling, the wall, and the floor. Several thousand feet of wire of different sizes are necessary. In addition, the power supply from the hospital's electrical transformer vault must be adequate. Custom-built shelving, work benches, and drawers will greatly facilitate the ease with which supplies can be made available. The nature of the x-ray equipment used requires adequate ceiling heights—a minimum of 9 feet 6 inches to the false ceiling. The lighting in the room should be of incandescent type and should be controlled with resistors allowing adjustment of light level. Piped-in suction apparatus and oxygen are desirable. Wiring from auxiliary apparatus, such as the electronics monitoring system with its leads, should be in the floor to the table base, thereby permitting the application of the leads to the patient without cluttering the area around the table with unnecessary surface wiring.

The minor surgery room should be equipped with operating lights, sterilizer, sinks, and the usual equipment found in a minor surgery room. The laboratory should have equipment permitting careful and adequate blood studies.

An improperly designed cardiac suite can contribute to unsuccessful examinations, whereas a carefully designed suite will contribute greatly to examination efficiency.

DIAGNOSTIC TEAM

During the course of a cardiovascular procedure it is not unusual for as many as twelve or fourteen people to be present in the room. Some of these are observers who are learning techniques; others constitute the basic team. Departments of radiology will vary in their approach to the members of the staff for this section of the department.

The first member of the team is the radiologist in charge of the examination. He is in control of the fluoroscopy and is directing a second member of the team, who may be a radiologist, a cardiologist, an internist, or, depending upon the type of examination being carried on, any other medical specialist. This second person is responsible for making the cutdown, exposing the vessel, and physically pushing the catheter into the desired areas under fluoroscopic direction from the radiologist. A third person is in charge of the monitoring systems. In some instances this will be a medical technician; in others, a resident physician. A medical technologist is present to perform laboratory examinations on the blood samples that are being extracted through the catheter during the procedure. The final members of the team are two x-ray technicians. Since we are primarily concerned with the duties of the x-ray technician in this book, their function in the cardiovascular procedure are described in detail.

X-RAY TECHNICIAN IN THE CARDIOVASCULAR SUITE

In the field of radiology, as well as in other medical specialties, there has been a trend toward specializing in a phase of the specialty. An x-ray technician with optimum skills in the basic fundamentals of the profession must acquire additional skills to become an expert cardiovascular x-ray technician. The calculated risks in these examinations allow no room for technical error.

The x-ray technician must understand and be able to apply a wide range of knowledge to help ensure the success of each procedure. He must be able to utilize his x-ray equipment to the fullest. This means proper selection of exposure factors, proper positioning of the patient, proper collimation of the x-ray beam, proper selection of film, proper selection of grids, and the ability to carefully evaluate each individual patient on the basis of the technical problems such a patient might present. The technician must have a calm, careful, and analytical attitude toward his duties. In preparing for each examination, a genuine understanding of the problems involved is necessary. A knowledge of the vocabulary used by the team is important.

The cardiovascular x-ray technician must acquire skills beyond those normally required for an x-ray technician. He must understand and be prepared to supply all necessary sterile instruments and supplies for any given examination. He must assume the duties of a circulating nurse during the procedure. A general knowledge of surgical instruments, suture materials, syringes, needles, and other equipment is necessary. During the course of the procedure, a technician is often called upon to occupy a position similar to that of the scrub nurse in an operating room. These duties must be understood.

The technician should have some knowledge of television from an operator's standpoint. A basic knowledge of movie cameras, their lenses, the film transport speed, and other technical knowledge of this field is helpful.

To better serve the physicians conducting the examination, the technician should know the anatomy of the circulatory system and the abnormalities that might occur in this system. In addition, the cardiovascular x-ray technician needs certain personality attributes. He is often the person who helps to reassure and comfort the patient during an examination. He is the "bridge" team member present and supplies skills, regardless of examination type.

The make-up of the balance of the team will vary with each type of examination.

VASCULAR RADIOGRAPHIC AND FLUOROSCOPIC EXAMINATIONS
Heart catheterization

Heart catheterization is a procedure in which a catheter is inserted into an artery or vein under fluoroscopic control and directed to the various chambers of the heart. Its purpose is to obtain samples of the blood from the chambers of the heart and to monitor the heart during this process. Many diagnoses can be made by heart catheterization alone. As a rule, however, selective angiography or cineradiography is done in connection with the heart catheterization.

Angiocardiography

Angiocardiography is an examination in which films are made of the great blood vessels and the heart following the introduction of a contrast medium through a catheter which has previously been inserted or through a needle placed in a blood vessel. The contrast medium may be opaque or radiolucent. At times carbon dioxide is used as the contrast medium. A wide variety of abnormalities can be pinpointed with the angiocardiogram that cannot be found with ordinary heart catheterization. The angiocardiogram is usually done with a rapid series of films being exposed in two planes following the injection of the medium. The best approach to this biplane examination is by utilizing two high-powered x-ray transformers: one to fire the tube for the lateral projection, and the other to fire a tube for the anteroposterior projection.

Coronary arteriography

Coronary arteriography is an examination of the coronary arteries following the injection of a contrast medium through a catheter which has been advanced to the proper position prior to injection of the dye. It is also a biplane rapid film examination or a cineradiographic examination. The purpose of the examination is to discover abnormalities in the coronary arteries.

Peripheral arteriovenography

Peripheral arteriovenography is an examination of the peripheral circulatory system, particularly of the arms or legs. Ordinarily the films are made in a single plane, again following the injection of contrast medium, either through a catheter that has previously been placed or through a needle into a selected artery or vein. This study also is for the purpose of outlining abnormalities in arteries and veins.

Abdominal aortography

As the name indicates, abdominal aortography is an examination performed to discover disease or abnormalities in the abdominal circulatory system. The contrast material may be injected through a catheter placed in the aorta by the way of a femoral artery, directly injected by needle into the aorta (translumbar puncture), or injected intravenously. The intravenous method is used most often in elderly patients and in those who have known sclerotic disease.

The intravenous method, however, presents a somewhat different technical problem than occurs when an arterial injection is used. Because the contrast medium enters the venous system first, time must elapse before filming begins. The contrast-laden blood will require from 8 to 15 seconds or more to reach the point of interest, the arterial system. A gradual dilution of the agent will occur during this time period. Films of the right contrast are more difficult to obtain, since the difference in densities to be demonstrated is less than if the medium were directed directly into the aorta. The exposure factors used must ensure long-scale contrast.

A biplane abdominal aortogram present some technical problems which exist with other biplane studies but which are more troublesome in the abdominal area. Due to the density of the part under examination, a larger volume of secondary radiation occurs than would, for instance, be true in a biplane angio-cardiogram. This tends to cause fogging of the films, particularly in the antero-posterior projection. The scattered radiation fog is the result of secondary radiation generated from the patient. There are many methods of controlling, to some extent, this interference with film quality. One is to use a slower x-ray film in the film changer being used in the anteroposterior projection. A second helpful method is to fire the x-ray tubes alternately rather than simultaneously, with no film in the exposure path of the anteroposterior unit when the lateral tube is firing.

Aortoarteriography

Aortoarteriography is an examination in which a series of films is made of the abdomen and as much as possible of the lower extremities. Peripheral arteriovenography and abdominal aortoarteriography require larger than stand-dard-sized film. This examination is one of the reasons that a vascular radio-graphic suite must have adequate ceiling heights. The focal-film distance required to cover the area of interest is in excess of 5 feet. This extended focal-film distance allows coverage of an area up to 36 inches in length. The basic ap-proach to the examination is similar to that of the other vascular radiographic procedures. A contrast medium is injected, either through a needle or through a catheter, to opacify both the abdominal aorta and the blood vessels in the lower extremities. Ideally, the equipment should permit a shift of the table top during the film series. The completed examination results in a series of films covering the abdominal aorta and the femoral circulation. With the table shift, the patient is moved so that the lower part of the lower extremities is in the radiation field and the final films are of the arterial circulation in the lower leg, including the ankle. In each single exposure the x-ray technician is dealing with an area of the patient that has widely different densities. To produce a film of continuous quality over this range of patient density, it is necessary to use a filtering system in the aperture of the x-ray tube. The technique is established to produce proper density for the abdominal aorta. A stepless aluminum filter, gradually increasing in thickness, is introduced into the tube aperture running the long axis of the patient. This results in films of uniform quality throughout areas of varying patient density.

Carotid arteriography

Carotid arteriography is similar in method of approach to cerebral angio-graphy. It is done, however, for a different purpose. A needle is introduced into the carotid artery, and the patient is positioned and the exposure factors are arranged to cover the blood vessels in the neck as the contrast flows toward the head. This examination is performed to disclose abnormalities in the blood vessels of the neck, whereas cerebral angiography is performed to discover pathology existing in the brain. The carotid angiogram should be a biplane film in order to pinpoint the area in question for the surgeon who is to perform corrective surgery if there are positive findings.

Splenoportography

Splenoportography is an examination made for the purpose of studying the spleen, the liver, and the blood vessels supplying this area. This examination differs from other vascular studies in that the agent is introduced directly into an organ rather than into a vessel. A needle is passed through the abdominal wall into the spleen. The contrast agent is injected, which then flows into the veins of the upper abdomen. Technical factors and positioning are very similar to those used in aortography.

Renal angiography

Renal angiography might be called a subclassification of aortography, except in this instance the purpose of the examination is to evaluate the renal circulation only. The films are often made in two planes, and therefore the precautions necessary in biplane aortography must be observed.

The Rashkind technique

The Rashkind technique is a method involving the insertion of a catheter in the usual heart catheterization methods. In this instance, however, the catheter itself attacks the anomaly and in successful cases cures the condition without surgery. When the catheter is in a proper position, the tip is inflated and, in fact, is used as a sort of wedge.

Pacemaker

The pacemaker is a device for giving electrical stimulation to the heart and is used in chronic heart conditions of various kinds. The installation of pacemakers again involves catheterization and a surgical approach. This procedure is carried on in cardiovascular x-ray suites. The pacemaker is installed surgically under x-ray control.

A patient who has had the pacemaker installation will then lead a comparatively normal existence with this electrical device stimulating his heart.

Because the pacemaker is an electrical device and because it is installed in the patient, a complication occurs that becomes an emergency if the device breaks or becomes inoperative. Again, the unit is repaired or replaced under fluoroscopic control.

Other procedures

There are many other procedures in the vascular field that involve x-ray technicians and x-ray facilities, and it is probable that this field will continue to expand. The position of cardiovascular fluoroscopy and radiography is not at present clearly defined as far as the experimental transplants of the heart are concerned. However, as skills and techniques improve in this area, both in connection with the live transplantations of hearts as well as the introduction of artificial hearts, there is little question that the skills of the special procedure x-ray technician will be called upon for a contribution.

IMPORTANCE OF VASCULAR RADIOGRAPHIC AND FLUOROSCOPIC EXAMINATIONS

During the past few years, spectacular progress has been made in heart and blood vessel surgery due to advanced surgical techniques. The technician should have a general knowledge of the various surgical operations in order to understand the importance of his work. A few reasons for performing vascular radiographic and fluoroscopic procedures and the operations made possible by the information gained from them follow.

The renal angiogram often discloses abnormalities which are correctable by blood vessel surgery. In many persons, particularly those in the young middle-aged group, hypertension is a result of abnormal renal circulation. With proper diagnostic information, the surgeon is able to correct these abnormalities, which, if left unattended, could result in the patient's having a stroke or other difficulties. We are all familiar with the great strides made in heart surgery for the correction of many congenital as well as acquired defects. The diagnosis of diseased coronary arteries by coronary angiography and the development of surgical techniques for correction have resulted in advances in this area of cardiovascular surgery. Traumatic injury to the various blood vessels, which in the past usually resulted in death, can be corrected surgically in some instances. Vascular radiographic and fluoroscopic procedures are the principal tool in diagnosing these injuries. Dissecting aneurysms, which were fatal a few years back, are also responding to the combination of these diagnostic procedures and surgical correction. The solution of all of these cardiovascular problems requires a team of persons with diverse skills. The x-ray technician who is skilled in vascular radiographic and fluoroscopic procedures is not the least member of the team.

USE OF CONVENTIONAL X-RAY EQUIPMENT DURING SOME RADIOGRAPHIC AND FLUOROSCOPIC PROCEDURES

Heart catheterization, angiocardiography, cineradiography, and carotid arteriography can best be done with special equipment similar in kind to that described in this chapter. Some of the vascular radiographic examinations, however, can be done without special equipment or with simple modifications of standard equipment. Translumbar aortography, splenoportography, and some types of peripheral arteriovenous studies are in this category. If one or two films, made after injection of a contrast agent, are enough to supply the needed information, the examination can be made using standard x-ray units. The precautions, from an emergency standpoint, have to be observed. Sterile packs, suc-

Text continued on p. 190.

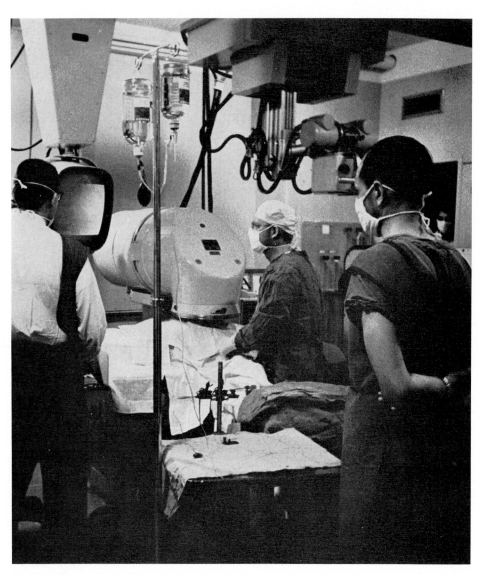

Fig. 9-1. Heart catheterization in progress.

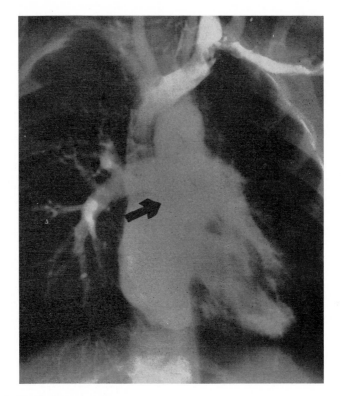

Fig. 9-2. Single film from angiogram.

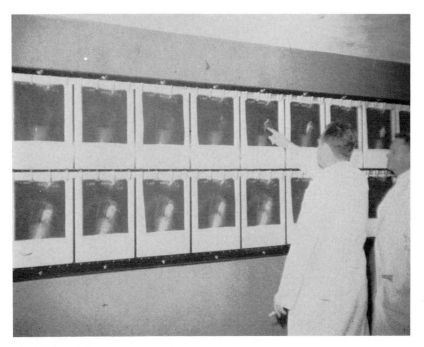

Fig. 9-3. Radiologist studying angiogram series.

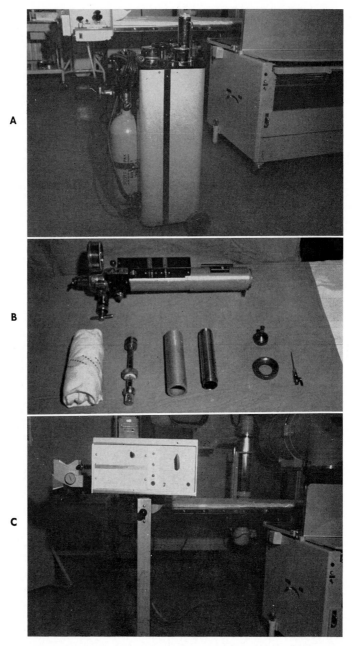

Fig. 9-4. Types of automatic injectors. **A,** Gidlund syringe. **B,** Amplatz syringe. **C,** Cordis syringe.

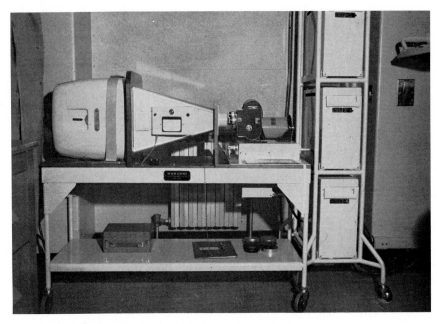

Fig. 9-5. Television monitor with cineradiography camera in place.

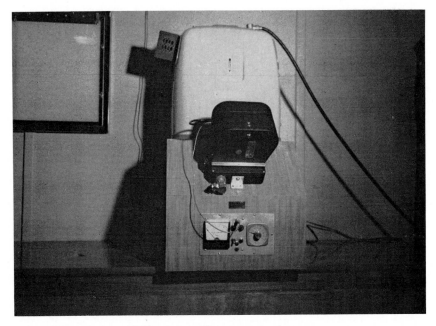

Fig. 9-6. Television monitor with 70 mm. spot film camera in place.

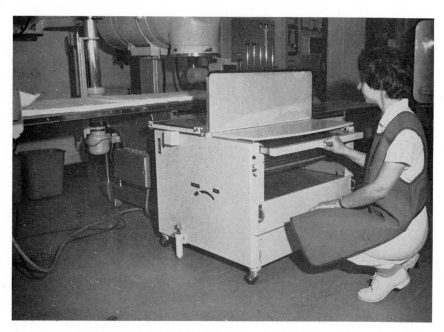

Fig. 9-7. Aortoarteriography table.

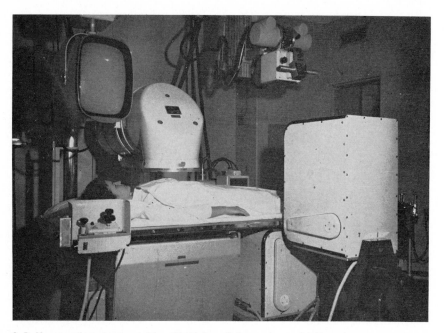

Fig. 9-8. Heart catheterization table with biplane Schonander rapid film unit.

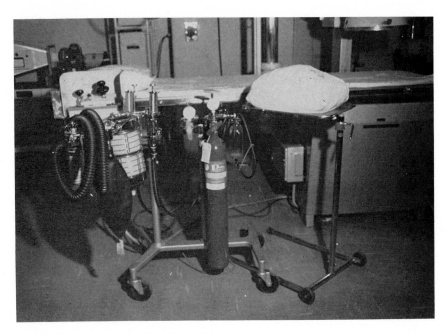

Fig. 9-9. Oxygen equipment and sterile pack.

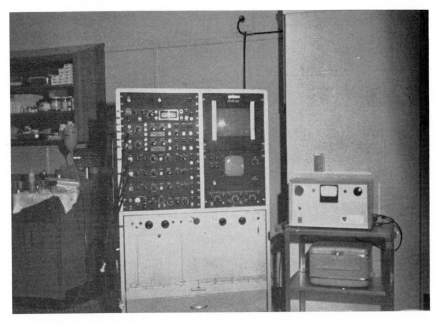

Fig. 9-10. Electronic monitoring equipment and defibrillator.

tion apparatus, oxygen equipment, and associated emergency apparatus should be available for immediate use.

Figs. 9-1 to 9-10 illustrate and describe typical cardiovascular suite equipment.

PREVENTION OF COMPLICATIONS WHICH MIGHT OCCUR IN THE VASCULAR EXAMINATIONS

There are many potential hazards that must be kept in mind by the technician in all types of vascular procedures. Sterile precautions must be observed at all times. The radiologic technologist in the cardiovascular suite is, in effect, also a scrub nurse. She must prepare the puncture site, for example, by seeing that it is shaved, if necessary, and cleansed. Following this preparation, an antiseptic solution must be applied and then the area draped with a sterile towel. When the sterile field has been prepared, great care must be exercised to see that this field is not inadvertently contaminated. The mass of equipment that is used in most of the procedures makes it difficult to avoid touching the sterile field with some piece of equipment unless constant vigilance is maintained.

The catheters and the equipment should always be in good operating condition. Absolute sterility of some of the equipment must be maintained. The catheters must not become clogged with foreign material or blood. A common complication in the vascular procedures is that the patient, following the procedure, may have a pyrogenic reaction. A pyrogen is protein organic matter of a fever-producing nature. When a patient has a pyrogenic reaction, it is a sign that the preparation of the catheters and auxiliary apparatus used in heart catheterization has been faulty. The transducer, the injector, the catheters—if nondisposable catheters are not being used, and other apparatus that is used to introduce the contrast medium through the catheter into the circulatory system is usually the suspected site for pyrogen.

Unless the equipment is very carefully cleansed and flushed immediately following use and before sterilization, there is a chance that a pyrogenic reaction can occur even if all equipment has been carefully sterilized. It is of extreme importance that proper procedure in cleansing the equipment following the examination is carried on.

Inspection of the catheters and the guide wires that are used within the catheters should be carefully made to determine whether any flaking or fraying is occurring. The guide wires should be flexible and should be inspected for flaws that might cause them to break. Any needles that are to be used during the procedure should be kept free of clots, and their ends should be inspected for burrs. The use of disposable products has helped to eliminate many of these problems.

Many solutions will be employed during the course of the vascular examinations. These include antiseptic solutions for preparing the skin of the patient, local anesthetics, saline for flushing catheters, and some drugs such as heparin, which is frequently used with the saline to prevent blood clotting, and finally, the contrast material which is to be injected with the pressure injector or, in some instances, with the hand injector. Great care to maintain the sterility of these solutions must be employed, and these materials, of course, must be properly identified on the tray.

At the end of a procedure after the catheter is withdrawn or the needle was withdrawn, pressure is applied over the vessel to prevent bleeding. If the puncture has been made in a vein, pressure is applied directly over the puncture site for several minutes. If the puncture is made in an artery, the pressure should be applied slightly above the puncture site and for a considerably longer period of time than would be necessary for a venous puncture. After releasing the pressure, the extremity should be checked to determine whether bleeding or any swelling that might indicate an accumulation of blood beneath the skin has occurred. If the extremity is cold or white or if the patient complains of pain, the physician should be notified.

Emergencies do arise during vascular procedures. They may range from a mild form of allergic reaction to the contrast medium to a complete cardiac arrest. Equipment to deal with this kind of emergency should be easily accessible to the cardiovascular suite, and the technician should know the location and use of this equipment.

REFERENCES

1. Cullinan, J. E.: The role of the x-ray technician in the cardiopulmonary laboratory, X-ray Technician **31**:623-628, 1960.
2. Dotter, C. T., and Steinberg, I.: Angiocardiography, Annals of Roentgenology, Series of Monographic Atlases, vol. 20, New York, 1951, Paul B. Hoeber, Inc., pp. 1-112.
3. Elliot, F. C., and Winchell, P.: Heart catheterization and angiocardiography, Amer. J. Nurs. **60**:1418-1422, 1960.
4. Gladden, J. L.: Angiocardiography, X-ray Technician **24**:330, 1953.
5. Gordon, J. J., Brahms, S. A., and Sussman, M. L.: Visualization of the coronary circulation during angiocardiography, Amer. Heart J. **39**:114, 1950.
6. Ide, A. W.: Venography of the deep veins of the thigh with a discussion of surgical applications, Thesis submitted to Faculty of the Graduate School of the University of Minnesota, 1951.
7. Kelly, A. E., and Gensini, G. G.: Coronary arteriography, Amer. J. Nurs. **62**:86-93, 1962.
8. Kelly, T. J.: The technician and angiocardiography, X-ray Technician **25**:11, 1954.
9. Lehman, J. S.: The technique of angiocardiography and thoracic aortography, X-ray Technician **24**:339, 1952.
10. Merrill, V.: Atlas of roentgenographic positions, ed. 3, St. Louis, 1967, The C. V. Mosby Co.
11. Meschan, I.: Roentgen signs in clinical diagnosis, Philadelphia, 1956, W. B. Saunders Co., chap. 22.
12. Moniz, E., deCarvalho, L., and Lima, A.: Angiopneumongraphie, Presse méd. **39**:996, 1931.
13. Morgan, R. H.: Problems of angiocardiography, Amer. J. Roentgen. **64**:189, 1950.
14. Olden, R. A.: Cinefluorography, X-ray Technician **33**:163-176, 1961.
15. Peddie, G. H., and Brush, F. E.: Cardio-vascular surgery—a manual for nurses, New York, 1961, G. P. Putnam's Sons.
16. Reich, N. E.: Diseases of the aorta, New York, 1949, The Macmillan Co., chap. 10.

17. Rigler, L. G.: Outline of roentgen diagnosis, Atlas Edition, Philadelphia, 1938, J. B. Lippincott Co., sec. D.
18. Robb, G. P.: An atlas of angiocardiography, American Registry of Pathology, Armed Forces Institute of Pathology, 1951.
19. Robb, G. P., and Steinberg, I.: Visualization of the chambers of the heart, the pulmonary circulation, and the great blood vessels in man: Practical method, Amer. J. Roentgen. 41:1, 1939.
20. Roesler, H.: Clinical roentgenology of the cardiovascular system, ed. 2, Springfield, Ill., 1946, Charles C Thomas, Publisher.
21. Starch, C. B.: Fundamentals of clinical fluoroscopy, New York, 1951, Grune & Stratton, Inc., chap. 3.
22. Stroud, W. D.: Diagnosis and treatment of cardiovascular disease, ed. 4, Philadelphia, 1950, F. A. Davis Co., chap. 52.
23. Sussman, M. L., Steinberg, M. F., and Grishman, A.: Multiple exposure technique in contrast visualization of the cardiac chambers and great vessels, Amer. J. Roentgen. 46: 745, 1941.
24. Taylor, H. K., and McGovern, T.: Angiocardiography: anatomy of the heart in health and disease, Radiology 43:364, 1944.

Chapter 10

Radiography in the operating room and the recovery room

GENERAL CONSIDERATIONS

Originally operating room radiography was confined to fracture cases and an occasional film of the abdomen in search of a missing sponge. In recent years, however, there has been an increasing number of radiographic examinations carried on in the operating room where the calculated risk of using x-ray equipment is overcome by the benefit to be gained in the treatment and diagnosis of the patient's condition. In addition to radiography used in orthopedic surgery and the sponge search, cholangiography is now done during the course of gallbladder surgery when both patency and the presence of stones in the ducts must be determined. Radiography of the urinary tract during cystoscopy, the use of x-ray in open angiography and ventriculography are further examples of the types of procedures to be carried on in the operating room in recent years.

THE OPERATING SUITE
Physical plan

The operating suite is generally composed of induction rooms where the patient, through anesthesia, is gradually brought to a certain degree of unconsciousness; several operating rooms where the surgery is done; a postanesthesia recovery room where, immediately following surgery, the patient is cared for by a highly trained staff; several rooms where clean and sterile supplies and instruments are stored; plaster rooms; sterilizing rooms; a room where rubber gloves are prepared; utility rooms; scrub rooms; and the offices and dressing rooms of the personnel.

Medical asepsis

Medical aseptic techniques should be scrupulously carried out in all parts of the operating suite. Great care should be taken to prevent bacteria from being carried from the rest of the hospital into the suite by a soiled uniform, soiled shoes, uncovered hair, or a dirty or dusty portable x-ray machine. The technician should make very certain the machine, her uniform, shoes, and person are clean. In some operating suites, when the technician reports to the charge nurse or operating room supervisor, she will be given a clean gown and cotton "boots" to put on over her own uniform and shoes. A cotton cap to cover the hair and a mask to put on before entry into the operating room itself will always be provided as further aids in *medical* asepsis.

Surgical asepsis

Surgical asepsis, of course, is an integral part of the operating suite in the preparation of supplies and instruments used for the patient and in the techniques used by the operating team during surgery. It is important for the technician to know the areas of the operating room itself in order that surgical asepsis may be carried out and contamination prevented (Fig. 10-1).

The **sterile area** is the operative area. It includes the patient, the drapes, the surgeons, the scrub nurses, the small instrument tables, and finally the so-called "back table," which is sterile but apart from the operative field. Neither the technician nor the x-ray machine must ever touch any part of this area.

The **anesthesia area** includes the nurse-anesthetist or the physician-anesthetist and all the various tanks of gases at the head of the patient. This area

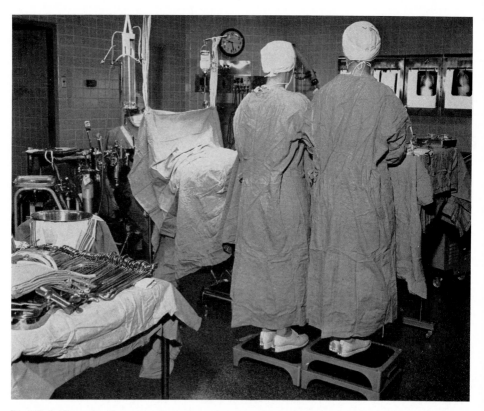

Fig. 10-1. The operating room. The two scrub nurses, the patient draped and in position, the instrument tables, and the "back table" are part of the sterile area. Note the anesthesia area and the nonsterile area with the patient's films on display. (Courtesy University Hospitals, Minneapolis, Minn.)

is not sterile. It is separated from the operative field by a high drape making a cotton wall between the patient's head and the operative site.

The nonsterile area includes the remainder of the room with the exception of the "back table." The circulating nurses, observers, and technicians move in this area only. Here is the view box where the patient's x-rays are posted and can be referred to during the surgery. The outlet for the x-ray machine is in this area, too. Because of the higher voltage necessary for the machine, the outlet may be different from those for other electrical equipment, having either a twist lock plug or one with an unusual shape.

HAZARDS IN THE OPERATING SUITE

A great deal of consideration is given to the hazard of possible explosion in operating suites where any spark could cause ignition of the highly volatile gases used in anesthesia. Many precautions are taken in an attempt to decrease or eliminate the possibility of spark formation. Since every person and thing has an electric potential or charge, it is of prime importance to equalize these charges so that no sparks are created. When the electric potential is different between two objects and the objects touch, there is a transfer of charge from the object of higher potential to the one of lower potential and a spark is created.

General precautions

Operating room wearing apparel receives attention, since cotton material has a low electric potential while the synthetic fabrics and wool have a higher charge. For this reason, uniforms of Dacron, nylon, or other synthetics are not worn in operating areas. Even nylon hose and underwear are not permitted in some hospital operating suites. The technician will have to gauge the type of apparel to be worn and follow whatever rules that have been instituted by the safety engineers in the hospital of employment. The aforementioned cap, placed over the hair, not only prevents bacteria spread from the hair but also cuts down static electricity. For this reason, too, wool blankets are not used in the operating room.

The control of temperature and humidity is a further precaution in equalizing electric potential, thereby reducing the possibility of spark formation. A cold, dry atmosphere increases the electric potential and, therefore, operating suites are kept warm and fairly humid.

It is necessary to check portable x-ray equipment before entry into the operating suite for medical asepsis and for the speedy completion of the technician's work. Moreover it behooves the technician to recognize any defects in the machine, thus preventing a possible explosion in the event there were a short in the apparatus. Observation of the "no smoking" rule is essential also.

Precautions in operating suite construction

A recent and logical trend toward further elimination of electrical hazards is in operating room construction. Extreme measures are being taken to make operating suites "explosion proof." In many institutions all electrical current to operating rooms comes from an isolated transformer source located outside of the operating room area. This type of transformer is nongrounded and is used for supplying the operating room area only. Assuming the *power source* has no leads to ground, the tendency then within the operating room is to use entirely nongrounded electrical medical equipment, such as operating room lights, surgical cutting units, suction machines, view boxes, and other apparatus. An operating room of this design has a conductive floor with electrical resistance built into it. The floor then acts as a drain for any static electricity that might be present within the operating room.

In hospitals where there is not a transformer or floor of this type or where the operating rooms are not of this design, precautions are taken to ground all equipment. Rubber casters are used on the portable x-ray machine to insulate the charge between equipment and the floor. Shoes must be free of lint and dirt, not only for sanitary reasons but also because lint and dirt act as conductors between the shoes and the floor and could create a spark. This is another reason some hospitals insist that technicians wear the aforementioned "boots" while in the operating area. All of these factors are further reasons why the portable x-ray machine should be checked for cleanliness before it is taken into the operating suite, since lint, thread, and accumulation of dirt act as conductors between the machine and the floor.

THE PATIENT, THE SURGICAL TEAM, AND THE TECHNICIAN
The patient

Occasionally the technician may have the opportunity of talking to the patient before he is anesthetized. The technician may be called to measure the patient, position him, and place the Bucky before he is draped. Every thoughtful consideration must be given him, realizing his natural fear and anxiety over the forthcoming surgery and that the operating room itself may appear awesome and startling. A quiet reassurance, careful handling, and a warm smile can mean much to him.

The technician should remember, too, that every operating room radiograph is considered an emergency. The film must be taken and developed as quickly as possible since the wound is open, the risk is great, and so is the cost to the patient for his being in the operating room. On the other hand, it is wrong to take and develop films in haste without regard to or at the risk of sacrificing quality. Such actions necessitate a second radiograph with greater risk and cost to the patient.

The surgical team

There may be several surgeons operating upon the patient with one or more doing the major surgery and one or more holding clamps, retractors, and assisting. They are highly qualified physicians who have specialized in the field of surgery.

The nurse who hands the surgeon instruments, sponges, needles, and sutures and generally assists him is called a scrub or an instrument nurse. Some types of surgery require more than one scrub nurse.

The surgeons and scrub nurses, wearing caps and masks, must wash and scrub their hands and arms well for 10 minutes. They then are assisted into sterile gowns and, avoiding contamination with anything unsterile, are helped on with the sterile gloves. They drape the patient and are the ones directly involved in the surgery.

The circulating nurses wear masks and caps, too, but these nurses are not "sterile." They circulate in the unsterile area, adjust the suction machines, intravenous feedings, and, using sterile forceps, hand the scrub nurse or surgeon anything required for the surgery that is not immediately available to them.

If the anesthesia is administered by a nurse who has taken special training in anesthesia, this person is called an anesthetist. If administered by a physician who has specialized in anesthesia, this person is an anesthesiologist. He carefully watches the patient's condition during surgery, selects various gas mixtures for certain types of patients and surgery and for various levels of anesthesia. He keeps an accurate record of the patient's blood pressure, his pulse and fluid intake, and his general response to the surgery. He takes and records the patient's vital signs every few minutes.

It is very necessary that the entire surgical team be aware of the hazards which are introduced with the use of x-ray equipment during the course of a surgical procedure. They must understand the complications involved, positioning required, and the needs of the x-ray technician in order to make it a safe, rapid, and effective procedure.

The technician

The very nature of operating room radiography makes certain demands upon the technician above and beyond those required for departmental or portable radiography. The technician must have a knowledge and understanding of operating procedures and the radiography required so that he or she can properly fit into the operating team without creating hazards to the patient due to ignorance of rules and techniques of surgical asepsis. The technician must be a mechanically adept person, since the x-ray machine and its maneuverability has to be substituted for the usual maneuverability of the part to be radiographed. Operating room radiography calls for a highly skilled person, too, with a thorough knowledge of the x-ray equipment to be used so that no need for repeat examinations is necessary. The technician must be of even temperament, able to function in an often tense atmosphere and to maintain composure and effectiveness despite pressures at the critical moments. The technician must obtain safely the proper radiograph under the existing conditions. Anything that might cause distraction from this objective must be ignored until the examination has been successfully completed and the patient's welfare ensured.

Radiographic procedure and technique

Having been summoned to the operating suite and regarding the work as emergent in nature, the technician should thoroughly check the portable x-ray machine for cleanliness and proper working order. Just as in portable radiography, the technician must report to the charge nurse in the operating suite in order to be directed to the correct room; be given any specific instructions regarding technique or patient care; and be given a clean cap, mask, and gown, not sterile ones.

Care must be taken when wheeling the portable machine into the operating room that no electrical equipment that is plugged in be disturbed. To unplug any suction or cautery machine, either by accident or in order to plug in the portable machine, can be very dangerous. The cords should not be run over by the machine, but lifted whenever possible.

Nearly all the x-ray work which is required during the course of surgery is somewhat complicated by the need for fast exposure time. Ideally this means that the x-ray equipment used in the operating room should have capacities comparable to fixed units available in the ordinary x-ray department.

In older hospitals where explosion-proof conditions are not possible, conventional portable x-ray equipment is usually used. In more recently constructed hospitals the entire operating room suite will be of explosion-proof construction. Making the operating rooms safe electrically is accomplished by creating a sparkproof area. The floors of the suite are of a conductive material with built-in electrical resistance. The floor acts as an electrical drain field. Personnel in the area must wear special shoes of a conductive material. All electrical apparatus is isolated from ground.

The evolution of electrically safe operating room areas has resulted in the development of explosion-proof mobile x-ray units. Any x-ray unit, during the course of exposure, may build up a static charge on the framework of the machine. This phenomenon is caused by the high voltages used. Normally the x-ray equipment is grounded, causing the electrical charge to travel to ground. An explosion-proof unit has a gas or airtight housing encasing the machine. By creating a different pressure inside the housing in relationship to the air in the room, any static charge is contained.

OPERATING ROOM PROCEDURES REQUIRING RADIOGRAPHY
The sponge search

The gauze sponges used during the course of surgery have a string or wedge of barium introduced into the weave. A major responsibility of the scrub or instrument nurse is keeping accurate count of the sponges used during surgery. If a short count is determined toward the completion of the operation, it becomes necessary to take a radiograph of the area in which the sponges have been used, to make sure that the missing sponge is not left within the patient. This complication may occur during abdominal surgery and the procedure will therefore require a film of the abdomen. A surgical sponge in itself has very little opacity and therefore will not cast a significant shadow when superimposed over thicker abdominal or anatomical parts. However, the string or wedge of barium, which is a part of the weave, does have sufficient opacity to cast a shadow and the determination of whether or not a sponge has been left within the operative site is not difficult.

A sponge search x-ray film may very well be required in a surgical procedure in which no x-ray work has been *anticipated*. Because the patient is already draped and on the operating room table, the surgical team and technician are faced with the problem of introducing a cassette under him without contaminating the sterile field. Ordinarily this is best done by having the surgeons and the scrub nurses physically handle the patient and roll him on his side or lift him from the table without contaminating the sterile field in order to permit the technician to insert the cassette under him in the proper area. The technician then brings the x-ray tube over the operating room table, being very careful not to contaminate the area, and makes the exposure. Following radiography, the patient has to be manipulated again to permit the technician to remove the cassette for processing.

If the procedure is one in which x-ray work *has* been anticipated, the Bucky diaphragm or a wooden cassette holder will have been a part of the preparation of the operating table before the patient is brought to surgery. The patient will have to be moved only to ensure his position over the cassette. The scrub nurse lifts the drapes permitting the technician to reach under them and introduce or remove the cassette from the area.

During the making of any radiograph under these conditions, the breathing of the patient can be controlled by the anesthesiologist. It is therefore necessary for the technician to alert him when all preparations for the radiograph have been made. The anesthesiologist, in turn, controls the breathing of the patient, suspends it for the time necessary to make the exposure, and signals the technician at the proper time.

Orthopedic surgery

During the fixation of a fractured hip with the hip nail or pin, the method of choice for making radiographs requires the use of two mobile x-ray units. In this instance more than ever, the x-ray equipment must be thoroughly cleaned by the technician before it is brought to the orthopedic operating room. After the patient is under anesthesia but before he has been surgically draped, these two units are placed in proper position for making an anteroposterior radiograph and a lateral radiograph. The first films are taken before surgery is begun. The machine to be used for the lateral film will have its tube with a collimated beam introduced between the legs of the patient. Usually a cylinder cone is used for this purpose. Most orthopedic operating tables have cassette-holding devices as integral parts of the table. This device should be in place and pushed into the area just above the crest of the hip and at the proper angle to permit project-ing the hip onto the film. After the machine to be used for the anteroposterior projection has been carefully centered above the proper area, the technician will make the necessary exposure. These radiographs will be of great value to the orthopedic surgeon in giving him the picture immediately preceding opera-tion. It may be necessary for him to make several exposures following adjust-ment of the orthopedic equipment before actually draping the patient and pre-paring to surgically insert the nail.

Parts of the x-ray equipment will then be draped into the surgical field and become an integral part of the table for all intents and purposes for the balance of the operation. Prior to draping, care should be taken by the tech-nician to protect the gonads of the patient from radiation, particularly if the patient is under 30 years of age, a child, or a pregnant woman. This can best be done by proper position, proper coning, and the use of lead cloth material underneath the draped area.

The cassette-holding part of the table is so constructed that it is possible for the technician to get under the surgical drape while the scrub nurse lifts the drapes, thus permitting the insertion or extraction of the cassette being used for the anteroposterior projections. For the lateral film, the surgeon or the scrub nurse will hold a sterile pillowcase to receive the cassette to be used. The tech-nician then introduces the cassette into the pillowcase, being very careful to maintain sterile technique and not allow the cassette to touch the outside of the sterile pillowcase. Grid cassettes should be used, since the hip is ordinarily an area that sets up considerable secondary radiation.

Processing should be arranged to permit rapid viewing of the films, since the radiographs taken in the course of a hip fixation are extremely important and a proper surgical result is dependent upon them. Some institutions have used fluoroscopy for this purpose. This method will not be discussed here, since it is the opinion of the author that the radiation hazard to the patient and the personnel make this practice unsound unless the fluoroscopic unit used is of the recently developed portable image intensifiers.

Cholangiogram

Cholangiography in the operating room is a common procedure and also a very valuable one from the standpoint of the welfare of the patient. Usually the surgical team can anticipate beforehand the need for a cholangiogram during the gallbladder surgery. Since this is so, it is wise for the technician to be familiar with the operating room schedule and, prior to surgery, measure the patient, see that the Bucky is padded, and that the cassette is correct in size and placement. In this way proper technical factors can be anticipated prior to surgery. In the occasional case where cholangiography is decided on *after* surgery has begun, the technician may have difficulty in properly classifying the patient for the purpose of determining exposure factors. In this instance, reference

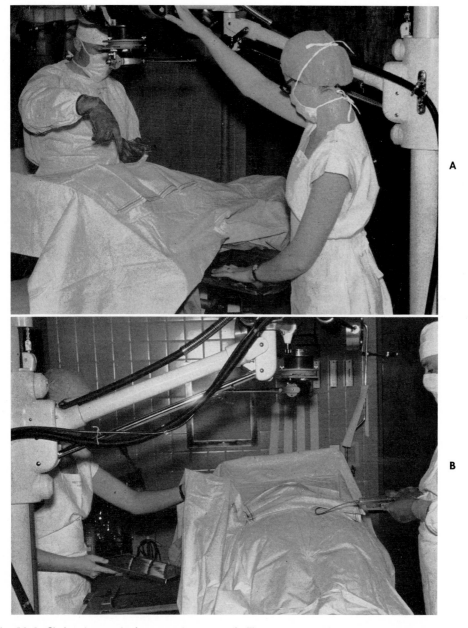

Fig. 10-2. Cholangiogram in the operating room. **A,** The surgeon is indicating the center point as the technician centers the x-ray tube. **B,** The technician has lifted the sterile drape to insert the cassette.

should be made to the patient's chart for his height, weight, and general build. With this information, the technician should then decide to take more than one film at the time of the cholangiogram, using slightly different factors in each film so that one of these will be of the proper diagnostic quality.

Ideally, the patient is positioned in such a fashion that the gallbladder and biliary duct area are over the film before surgery begins. The surgeon then proceeds with the operation and, after having removed the gallbladder, introduces a tube into the biliary duct. Teamwork is paramount in taking the cholangiogram. The surgeon covers the wound with a sterile towel. The technician centers the cone of the machine over the area. The surgeon and assistants help in alignment. The technician must be ready to manipulate the Bucky. The surgeon injects the dye. The anesthesiologist holds the patient's rebreathing bag, which constitutes holding the patient's breath, and signals "shoot." The resulting radiograph indicates the presence or absence of stones or other pathology in the biliary duct (Fig. 10-2).

Isolated kidney

Radiography of the kidney during the course of surgery is an occasional procedure required of the technician. This is necessary in some instances where the patient's kidney requires surgery but not removal. It means, therefore, that the technician must obtain a satisfactory radiograph of the kidney as it lies within the body. Certain problems exist in a procedure of this nature, since only the kidney is to be radiographed, and since the purpose of the radiograph is to determine whether the kidney is free of stones following the surgery that has been performed on it. Too, the film is to be introduced into the body cavity itself. It therefore becomes necessary to use a nonscreen container or a special cassette of a curved nature small enough to be introduced in the body, large enough to permit radiography of the entire kidney, and of a composition that permits sterilization. The simplest way to obtain a radiograph of this nature is to use film contained in a Manila envelope. The technician can obtain envelopes, usually 5 × 7 inches in size, and supply these to the nursing staff who, in turn, sees that they are autoclaved and included in the sterile supplies for this particular operation.

The technician should choose a film of sufficient size to obtain a radiograph of the entire kidney at one time and still be small enough to be fitted easily into the sterile Manila envelope. The film should be wrapped in black paper with a thin lead foil background in back of it. It is necessary to mark this paper-wrapped film since the lead side must be in back of the film in relation to the x-ray tube. The technician should bring several of these paper-wrapped films to the operating room.

The scrub nurse will hold the sterile envelope and the technician then carefully introduces the film into the sterile envelope, being careful to avoid contamination of the outer parts of the envelope. The envelope is then handed to the surgeon who lowers it through the incision into the body cavity and, at the same time, with the use of forceps, brings the kidney up in front of the film area as much as possible. The technician, by proper angulation of the tube, attempts to get as nearly as possible, a true projection of the x-ray beam through the kidney and to the film. The surgeon will then give the film to the technician who should handle it with care since the envelope, having been inside of the body, is covered with blood. Care must be taken in removing the film from the envelope to avoid contact with the blood. After processing, the resultant radiograph shows the presence or absence of stones and therefore helps determine the nature of the subsequent surgery.

Other procedures

There are, of course, many other x-ray procedures carried on in the operating room, such as ventriculography, open angiography, and cystoscopy. The procedures previously described, however, are the main types of examination. Others have the same radiographic complications and follow a similar radiographic procedure. They are also similar in the use of surgical asepsis.

Processing operating room radiographs

Normally, the films obtained during the course of surgery are of importance primarily at the time of operation. Their importance as part of the patient's over-all film record is not the same as those films which are made from time to time in the regular x-ray department. The fact that they are of immediate rather than later importance permits the use of processing procedures which normally should not be used in radiography. This is a matter of using special solutions which permit fast processing or using regular solutions beyond the normal developing temperatures. It is possible, for example, by heating the developer to the point of 80° or 85° F., to obtain film processing adequate for the immediate purpose in as little as 1 minute's time. Time spent in processing surgical x-ray procedures is of prime importance. In every instance the surgeon is awaiting the x-ray results. This means that the patient's abdomen or other area undergoing surgery is left open and that anesthesia is being continued. Both of these conditions contribute to surgical risk. It is of importance, and, in this instance, to a degree superseding the desire to attain radiographic quality, that the films be processed and returned to the surgeon with extreme speed. In some instances the operating room will have an adjacent darkroom. This, together with speed-up solutions, is probably the best answer to the processing problem in the operating room.

There are available small electrically heated processing units which can be used for the occasional operating room radiograph, thus permitting the surgeon to see films in as little as 2 or 3 minutes. Polaroid units are available also which utilize the dry processing method, making it possible to have exposed film available for viewing in less than a minute. This type of processing results in the film having poorer permanent quality but will very well answer the purpose at the time of the surgical procedure. In this respect, therefore, it is necessary for the technician to compromise permanent film quality in favor of speed processing.

THE RECOVERY ROOM

Within the last 15 years recovery rooms or intensive care units have found their place in the modern hospital, thus playing a great part in the advance of surgical procedures. New and dramatic types of surgery would often prove ineffective unless corresponding expert care was given during the immediate postoperative period when the patient is recovering from the anesthetic. Not many years ago, all surgical patients were returned immediately to their beds on the ward to be cared for by the regular medical team. The plan of providing a special recovery room in the operating room area, where patients can be watched over and cared for by a specially trained team of nurses, anesthesiologists, and surgeons, has proved highly successful.

Most recovery rooms have eight or ten beds where the surgical patient is cared for until his blood pressure no longer fluctuates and he is awake enough to swallow his own saliva and mucus, usually from 2 to 6 hours. Here facilities

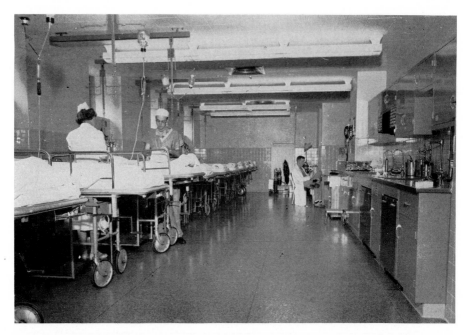

Fig. 10-3. The postoperative recovery room. Here the patient can receive expert care in the immediate period following surgery. The recovery room has ceiling mountings for intravenous bottles, piped-in oxygen, wall suction, a 220-volt receptacle for high-powered x-ray units between each stretcher, and emergency equipment available, all aiding in giving patient care. (Courtesy University Hospitals, Minneapolis, Minn.)

are provided for oxygen therapy, gastric suction, and chest suction. Emergency drugs and equipment for tracheotomy or cardiac massage are also available (Fig. 10-3).

With the advent of the recovery room has come an increased use of immediate postoperative radiography. In most instances this radiography is confined to the chest. The surgeons, nurses, and anesthesiologists are often dependent on the technician to help them determine whether the patient has developed some serious postoperative complication. When called to the recovery room, the technician must realize that this, too, is an emergency situation. This call should be placed above all others and the technician should do everything within his power to appear at the door ready to take the film within a few minutes. Usually, a maze of bustle and activity will greet the technician. Some patients may be responding and semiconscious; others may be completely unconscious. Many will be receiving parenteral fluids or nasal oxygen; some may have gastric suction or urinary catheters. An "airway" may be in the mouth of the surgical patient to keep the tongue forward and not interfere with breathing.

In the recovery room, radiographs of the chest are generally taken in a sitting position, for if there is any air in the chest cavity, it rises and will be more visible in this position. The problems of taking such a film are quite different from the ordinary chest procedure on the wards or in the main x-ray department. The specially trained recovery room nurse must participate in the examination to a greater degree than would be true in a conventional portable radiograph of the chest. Due to the complicated apparatus and the condition of the patient, the person with special training should be charged with positioning the patient. The technician's function is the arrangement of the x-ray equipment to compensate for any departure from ordinary in the positioning of the patient. The technician should have all technical factors ready so that when the signal is given, the backrest can be raised, the cassette slipped behind the patient's back so that he is leaning on it, and the film taken immediately before the patient can slip down out of position. The recovery room nurses hold the patient, but keeping him in one position for any length of time is impossible, since the unconscious patient is unable to do anything for himself. He cannot follow directions, he cannot understand, he cannot move by himself. Hence, there must be no delay and the taking of the radiograph must be like clockwork.

Again it is necessary to use fairly high capacity mobile x-ray equipment if these films are to be satisfactory. After a film has been taken in the recovery room, the technician's responsibility is not over. No time can be wasted in processing, because the patient's immediate future and the course of action of the surgeon is often dependent on what is visualized on the films.

Radiography in the recovery room truly involves teamwork. Cooperation between the staff and the x-ray technician can ensure adequate films. Each must be understanding of the other's problems, and the adjustment from normal procedure will have to be made by the x-ray technician in the best interest of the patient. A system and a technique are necessary whereby the unconscious and critical patient is cared for with skill and intelligence and without waste of time.

REFERENCES

1. Beach, R.: Electrostatic explosion controls in hospital operating rooms, J. Amer. Assoc. Nurs. Anes. **21**:143-145, 1953.
2. Bechtal, R. C. L.: What an orthopedic surgeon looks for in a roentgenogram, X-ray Technician **26**:334, 1955.
3. Berry, E. C., and Kohn, M. L.: Introduction to operating room technique, New York, 1955, Blakiston Div., McGraw-Hill Book Co., Inc.
4. Booth, S. C.: Recovery room service, Amer. J. Nurs. **51**:356, 1951.
5. Carnahan, J.: Recovery room for postoperative patients, Amer. J. Nurs. **49**:581, 1949.
6. Casper, S. L.: Principles of fracture roentgenography, X-ray Technician **24**:510, 1952.
7. Clark, B. G., Phillips, R. I., Goade, W. J., and Ettinger, A.: Recent advances in radiography of the urogenital organs, X-ray Technician **27**:175, 1955.
8. Cratens, J. E.: Physiology of the liver and gallbladder in relation to their radiographic study, X-ray Technician **15**:144-146, 1944.
9. Eliason, E. L., Ferguson, L. K., and Sholtis, L. A.: Surgical nursing, ed. 10, Philadelphia, 1955, J. B. Lippincott Co., chaps. 3, 5, 11, 18, 30, 31.
10. Felter, R. K., West, F., and Zetzsche, L. M.: Surgical nursing, Philadelphia, 1952, F. A. Davis Co., chap. 44.
11. Guest, P., Sikora, V., and Lewis, B.: Static electricity in hospital operating suites: direct and related hazards and pertinent remedies, Bulletin 520, Bureau of Mines, Washington, D. C., 1953, Government Printing Office.
12. Gulley, D. E.: Radiography of the exposed kidney, X-ray Technician **27**:193, 1955.
13. Harmer, B., and Henderson, V.: Textbook of the principles and practice of nursing, New York, 1955, The Macmillan Co., chap. 8.
14. Kerr, H. D., and Gillies, C. L.: The urinary tract: a handbook of diagnosis, Chicago, 1944, The Year Book Publishers.
15. Lesmeister, Sister Viola: Cholangiography, X-ray Technician **25**:346, 1954.
16. Lowsley, O. S., and Kerwin, T. J.: Urology for nurses, ed. 2, Philadelphia, 1948, J. B. Lippincott Co., chap. 5.
17. McGowen, J. H.: Radiography of the ventricular system of the brain, X-ray Technician **24**:14, 1952.
18. McMahon, J., and Fife, G.: Nursing problems in recovery room anesthesia, Amer. J. Nurs. **45**:618, 1945.
19. Merrill, V.: Atlas of roentgenographic positions, ed. 3, vol. 2, St. Louis, 1967, The C. V. Mosby Co.
20. Meschan, I.: Roentgen signs in clinical diagnosis, Philadelphia, 1956, W. B. Saunders Co., chap. 25.
21. National Fire Protection Association: Recommended safe practice for hospital operating rooms, Boston, 1952, The Association.
22. Rigler, L. G.: Outline of roentgen diagnosis, Atlas Edition, Philadelphia, 1938, J. B. Lippincott Co., sect. 9.
23. Sadove, M. S., and Cross, J.: Recovery room—immediate postoperative management, Philadelphia, 1956, W. B. Saunders Co.
24. Sante, L. R.: Manual of roentgenological technique, ed. 12, Ann Arbor, Mich., 1945, Edwards Bros., Inc., pp. 228-271.
25. Schafer, M. K., and Galbraith, T. P.: Recovery room services, Hospitals **26**:65, 1952.
26. Thomas, G. J.: Explosion hazards in operating and delivery rooms, J. Amer. Assoc. Nurs. Anes. **18**:26, 1950.

Chapter 11

Emergency receiving
x-ray procedures

GENERAL CONSIDERATIONS

An emergency may be defined as an unforeseen set of circumstances which call for immediate action. A medical emergency might result from a sudden onset of disease, a sudden change for the worse in an existing disease, or injury resulting from an accident. Most hospitals, except those of a highly specialized character, have an emergency receiving department. Emergencies have as a common characteristic an urgent need for treatment.

The staffing of an emergency area varies with the size of the case load to be admitted. The basic staff should include a competent physician and a nurse supervisor with specialized skills in emergency situations. A person in an administrative capacity who is capable of gaining the confidence of relatives or friends accompanying the patient is also necessary. Such a person is responsible for obtaining identification data, pertinent addresses, etc. Specially trained orderlies or attendants should be available. Various medical specialists should be on call at all times. A skilled x-ray technician should also be available. Routine and special procedure examinations on a patient admitted to an emergency receiving room often present technical problems markedly different from those encountered in a scheduled x-ray examination.

EMERGENCY CASE LOAD

A fairly high percentage of the patients admitted to an emergency receiving unit arrive there as a result of some type of accident. The remainder are admitted as a result of a sudden onset in illness or aggravation of an existing disease. Statistics reveal that there is a continuous upward trend in the number of patients being admitted to emergency receiving departments and that the use of the x-ray examination as a diagnostic tool is increasing at a faster pace than the case load.

A study of the records of two institutions revealed that in 1958 there was a request for one x-ray examination for every seven admissions, whereas in 1967, there was a request for one x-ray examination for every three and a half admissions. These statistics may not be representative of all hospitals, but they do emphasize a trend that is of concern to x-ray department personnel—that not only are more patients being admitted to emergency units who require x-ray examinations but that more x-ray examinations per patient are also required. As a result of this information, it behooves hospitals to have on their staff x-ray technicians who are skilled in emergency procedures and to plan the x-ray department to accommodate the increasing demand for x-ray examinations on the emergency service.

This, of course, will present problems: (1) x-ray departments will have to be staffed 24 hours a day, (2) x-ray training programs must produce x-ray technicians skilled in emergency procedures, (3) the emergency area, or the x-ray department if the emergency examinations are to be done there, must have equipment that will allow the flexibility necessary to make a good x-ray examination in spite of a considerable departure from routine exposure factors and positioning.

EMERGENCY RECEIVING ROOM X-RAY TECHNICIAN

It is not uncommon to find that much of the emergency x-ray work is being done by student technicians or inexperienced staff technicians. This is particularly true in after-hour staffing. This, of course, is a mistake in the approach to the best method of handling emergency x-ray procedures.

An x-ray technician doing emergency procedures not only must be basically well qualified, but he must also have the following skills and personal qualities:

1. Personality traits that allow careful work under extreme pressure
2. Ability to improvise positions when the condition of the patient does not permit routine positioning
3. Greater skills in the nursing arts than would commonly be expected of a registered x-ray technician
4. Rare professional judgment
5. Dedication to his profession

The referring physician in an emergency x-ray service may not be aware of the mechanics of positioning for various types of radiographic examinations. He must therefore rely on the technician to inform him of the positioning requirements of the x-ray examination requested. Then, if the condition of the patient is such that the view is unobtainable or is contraindicated, the physician can suggest another procedure.

EMERGENCY PATIENTS

Accident patients admitted to the emergency room of a hospital often present bizzare complications both to the physician, who, in most instances, is seeing him for the first time, and to the x-ray technician, who more often than not must adapt methods in order to obtain the best possible x-ray films for diagnostic purposes. The patient may have multiple injuries, some very obvious and some concealed. Often he will be in shock, which complicates the discovery of some of his injuries. He may have lacerations, fractures, internal as well as external bleeding, and rupture of internal organs. A principal problem is that the patient's medical history is not available to the physician in most instances. A percentage of these patients may have heart disease, diabetes, or some other chronic condition that possibly has been aggravated by the accident.

The physician in the emergency receiving area usually treats shock and controls bleeding before ordering x-ray examinations or laboratory procedures. When the patient is ready for x-ray examination, the mechanics of carrying on the procedures are often complicated by the fact that intravenous solutions or blood plasma is being administered. In some instances, temporary fixation devices for fractures have been applied. Some patients may be under the influence of alcohol or narcotics. Severely injured patients are usually comatose and noncooperative.

The patient admitted because of an emergency medical condition also presents a variety of problems. He may be suffering from any of a variety of ailments: ruptured peptic ulcer, acute heart failure, gallstone colic, renal colic, ingestion of poison, overdose of sleeping tablets, epileptic seizures, or a vascular accident. X-ray examinations for evaluation purposes may be ordered for these patients, and in many instances the examination cannot be made in a routine manner.

X-RAY EQUIPMENT FOR THE EMERGENCY RECEIVING AREA

A basic requirement for x-ray equipment used in emergency work is flexibility. The x-ray tube will have to be maneuvered into many angulations not

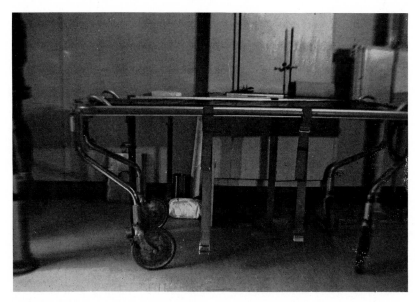

Fig. 11-1. Stretcher that is x-ray transparent with movable top to ease moving of the patient to x-ray table.

commonly used. It is essential that the tube can be securely locked in all of these positions. Since we are quite often dealing with noncooperative patients, it is necessary that the equipment be of high capacity. The x-ray timer on the unit should permit extremely fast exposure times at high milliamperage and kilovoltage.

The x-ray tables should be of a tilt type, equipped with suitable compression devices. A light portable x-ray unit should be included as part of the emergency room x-ray equipment. The emergency receiving area should be equipped with several special stretchers. These stretchers will differ from a routine type of hospital stretcher in that the top of the stretcher should be a material that is x-ray transparent. It will be helpful if the stretcher top is portable and easily removed from its carriage, such as that shown in Fig. 11-1. You will note that handles are attached to the stretcher top, making it possible to move the stretcher from its wheels to place the patient on an x-ray table without moving the patient himself physically. This feature, combined with a radiolucent table top, permits x-ray work through the top of the stretcher and, in some instances, through the x-ray table top to its Bucky diaphragm.

With the motor-driven x-ray table, it is possible to move the x-ray table into the vertical position. A patient lying on the stretcher may then be brought in front of the vertical table and the Bucky diaphragm can be utilized for cross-stretcher radiography, which is often necessary when the patient cannot be moved (Fig. 11-2).

The x-ray area in the emergency receiving unit should have the routine acces-

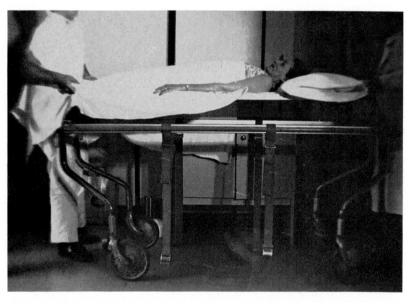

Fig. 11-2. An emergency patient being transferred to x-ray table without being physically moved.

sories common to all x-ray rooms. It is desirable also to have some additional specially constructed accessories. Cassettes with high-speed screens to assist in making a fast exposure time should be available. Grid cassettes for cross-table or cross-stretcher radiography are necessary and are used in many types of examinations. Emergency kits containing the drugs and instruments for use should be available in the event the patient's condition deteriorates while undergoing x-ray examination. For the same reason, suction apparatus and oxygen should also be available in the x-ray room. Since the films should be made available to the physician as quickly as possible, adequate darkroom facilities should be adjacent to the emergency x-ray area.

EMERGENCY X-RAY EXAMINATIONS

The technician must bear in mind that any accident may result in multiple injuries. He must be guided by the fact that a routine approach to any given examination may have an adverse effect on another part that is injured but not under immediate consideration. It would be very difficult to lay out a standard approach to each type of examination necessary in an emergency receiving area. Successful results are a matter of experience and good judgment on the part of the x-ray technician, coupled with adequate x-ray equipment. However, suggested approaches to representative emergency problems, such as those given below, should be helpful.

Examples of emergency receiving problems

Case 1. A patient is admitted in a comatose condition. The x-ray request disclosed a provisional diagnosis of fracture of the skull, possible fractured ribs, and a fracture of the femur. The referring physician wishes to have x-ray films of the skull and the chest and rib area. The fractured femur has been temporarily splinted and is not under immediate consideration. This patient is on a stretcher, and intravenous fluids are being administered. The x-ray problem in this case is to obtain a sufficient number of films of the skull to evaluate the skull for fracture. It is further necessary to obtain films of the chest area to determine whether fractured ribs have pierced the lungs. The complicating factor is that this person has a fracture of the femur which has been temporarily treated with a Thomas splint. In addition, the patient is in a comatose condition. This means that the usual approach to making a series of skull films, as well as the usual films of the rib area, is contraindicated. The skull examination and the chest examination must be made with an absolute minimum of movement of the patient.

Assuming that an x-ray–transparent stretcher (Fig. 11-1) is in use, the patient is carefully transported from the carriage of the stretcher to the x-ray table. Using a grid cassette, a left lateral skull film is made first (Fig. 11-3). Then, again with the grid cassette, the opposite lateral skull film is made (Fig. 11-4). Note that the flexibility of the equipment has permitted the making of these first two

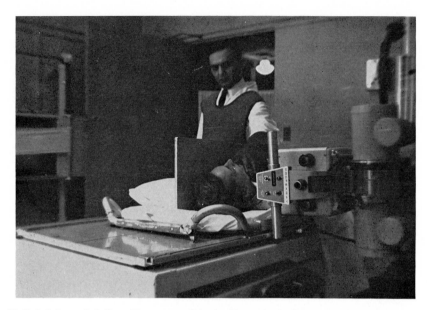

Fig. 11-3. Left lateral skull position accomplished without physically moving the patient.

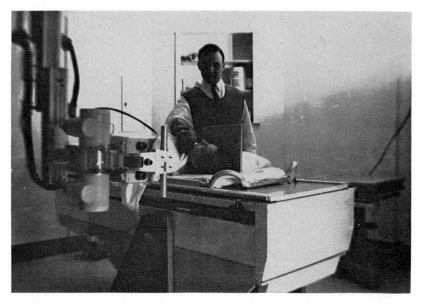

Fig. 11-4. Right lateral skull position accomplished without physically moving the patient.

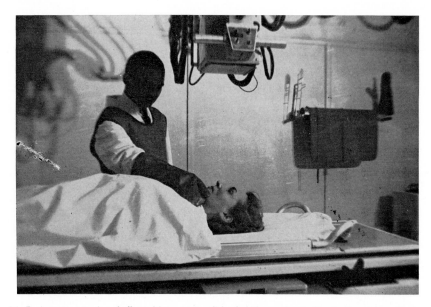

Fig. 11-5. Anteroposterior skull position accomplished without physically moving the patient.

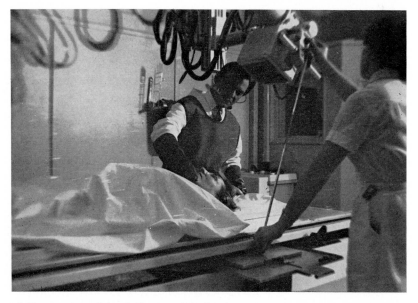

Fig. 11-6. Townes view of the skull accomplished without physically moving the patient.

films without any movement of the patient. To complete the skull portion of the examination, an anteroposterior projection of the skull is made, followed by one of the base of the skull, using the Townes view. These two projections are made through the transparent stretcher top and the top of the x-ray table, utilizing the x-ray table's Bucky diaphragm (Figs. 11-5 and 11-6).

A patient in a comatose condition will require some form of immobilization during exposure of the films. Extremely fast exposure times should be used. The most successful method of immobilizing the skull is to have an assistant, who is properly clothed in a lead apron and lead gloves, physically hold the patient's chin. By using careful collimation and by placing the person restraining the patient in the right location, this person will be prevented from receiving a significant amount of radiation (Fig. 11-7). An orderly, a nurse, or even a relative or friend who accompanied the patient can be used for this purpose. The use of nonradiologic personnel properly equipped with the lead protective garments is the simplest answer to the immobilization problem.

To complete the x-ray examination, the next step would be to make a single anteroposterior film of the chest area. This film also would be made with the cassette in the Bucky diaphragm and the x-ray beam penetrating the patient, the table top, and the transparent stretcher top. Utilizing this method will increase the part-film distance somewhat, since the stretcher top will also be between the patient and the cassette, in addition to the table top. It therefore is wise, assuming that the exposure factors are not compromised too greatly, to

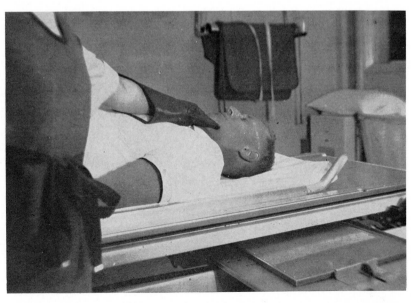

Fig. 11-7. Proper position of the hand of a person immobilizing the patient's head for a skull series.

take these films at an increased focal-film distance. The increased focal-film distance would tend to minimize the loss of sharpness occurring when an increased part-film distance exists. In making the chest-rib portion of this examination, the x-ray machine must be used in a fashion to give the fastest possible exposure time. A comatose patient is not going to be able to suspend respiration. The technician must watch carefully and attempt to make the exposure while the patient is in inspiration on the breathing cycle.

Evaluation of the films obtained should give the emergency room physician enough information to proceed with treatment. It will also provide necessary clues to the patient's condition to aid in determining whether it is possible to make further x-ray studies of a more complex nature. The films might disclose that it is no longer considered dangerous to position the patient into proper positions for additional films.

Case 2. A common medical emergency encountered in the emergency receiving areas is the patient with acute abdominal symptoms. In most instances these patients can be examined in the routine fashion using routine positions. Fairly often, however, the patient is too ill to stand. Acute abdominal symptoms have a wide variety of causes, and the emergency physician is handicapped by not having medical history. Some acute abdomen conditions dictate immediate surgery. The patient may have gallstone colic, renal colic, or a ruptured ulcer. Of importance in arriving at a diagnosis is the determination of whether or not there is fluid or free air in the abdominal cavity. The x-ray examination that best demonstrates this is a flat plate of the abdomen with the patient in the supine position, followed by an upright or a lateral decubitus film of the abdomen to demonstrate air or fluid levels. The upright films must include the diaphragm, since air will gather under the diaphragm.

Since these films cannot be made in the routine manner in the patient who is too ill to stand, the following procedure is suggested. A series of three films is indicated. First, conventional anteroposterior films of the abdomen are made with the patient lying on the table in a supine position. The film is centered to include the diaphragm and the pelvis. Compression devices are then fixed across the patient at the level of the buttocks and the chest. The footrest is installed at the bottom of the x-ray table. The table is then motor driven toward the vertical position under careful observation by the technician. When the table is at an angle of approximately 75° to 80°, it is stopped. At this point the patient is nearly upright but, due to the footrest and restraining devices, is in no danger of falling. After positioning the cassette to include the diaphragm, the technician should proceed to position the x-ray tube in a fashion that results in the x-ray beam being parallel with the floor (Fig. 11-8, A). Many technicians make the error of attempting to position the x-ray tube with an angle that compensates for the angle of the table. When this tube position is used, the resulting film is similar to that obtained on the original supine projection. If information regarding air or fluid is essential, it is of paramount importance to position the x-ray tube

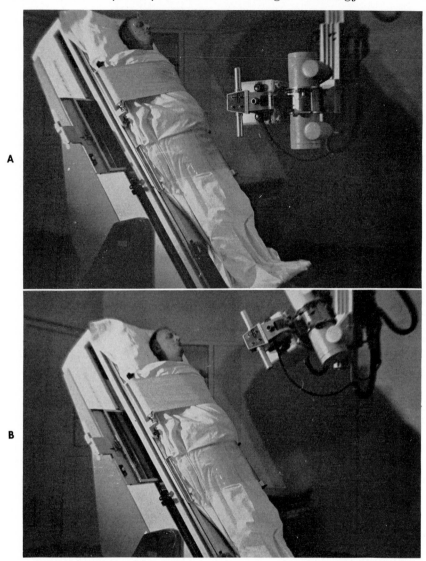

Fig. 11-8. A, Correct semierect position for films of the abdomen to demonstrate air or fluid levels. **B,** Incorrect semierect position for films of the abdomen to demonstrate air or fluid levels.

properly. See Fig. 11-8, *A,* for correct position and Fig. 11-8, *B,* for incorrect position. A third film, made without changing the position of the patient but rather by moving the cassette to include the pelvis, is helpful.

Case 3. With the steady increase in injuries resulting from automobile accidents, many emergency spine examinations are required. We are all familiar with the term "whiplash injury." This injury occurs frequently as the result of the sudden stop which occurs in an accident. Often x-ray examinations are requested

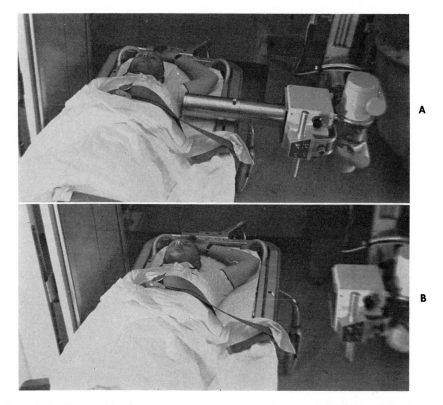

Fig. 11-9. A, Position used for first exposure to demonstrate the seventh cervical and the first and second thoracic vertebrae, accomplished without physically handling the patient. **B,** Preparing for second exposure after removing cone.

on a patient who has an injury to the spine, particularly to the cervical or upper thoracic spine. In routine radiography it is difficult to demonstrate the seventh cervical and first and second thoracic vertebrae successfully. In the emergency patient who has other injuries complicating the examination, this problem becomes more pronounced. In a suspected spine fracture, the patient should not be moved in any manner that normal positioning of this patient would require until it has been determined that no serious spine injury is present.

Assuming that an x-ray examination of the cervical and upper thoracic region is requested, the following procedure is suggested. Without removing the patient from the stretcher, place a grid cassette upright on the stretcher and position the x-ray tube to shoot across the stretcher. Position the cassette in a fashion to include the first and second thoracic and all seven cervical vertebrae. Insert a cylinder cone into position on the x-ray tube. Then extend the cone to cover the first and second thoracic and seventh cervical vertebrae (Fig. 11-9, *A*). Establish high penetration exposure factors at the x-ray control. Following the x-ray exposure, rapidly remove the cone, establish new routine lateral cervical spine exposure factors on the control, and repeat the exposure. This is done without moving the patient or the cassette. The resulting radiograph will have a double exposure, including a coned area over the difficult-to-obtain seventh cervical and first and second thoracic vertebrae. The balance of the film will include the rest of the cervical spine. This special technique is very useful in obtaining films of the cervical thoracic region particularly from a continuity standpoint. The films, of course, can be made without moving the patient (Fig. 11-9, *B*). It is wise to make a routine cross-table cervical spine film in addition to the special view.

Upon evaluation of the two films described, the physician can determine how to proceed with treatment. Assuming that a fractured vertebra is present, routine approach to the x-ray examination could have serious results. The positioning necessary might cause the fractured parts to impinge on the spinal cord, resulting in paralysis and permanent damage. Using the correct procedure, on the other hand, could contribute to eventual complete recovery.

Case 4. Another common but complicated type of an emergency x-ray examination is on the patient who has received multiple injuries to the facial bones. This type of injury is usually the result of a fight, a beating, or an automobile accident. It may or may not be complicated by the presence of other injuries.

We will assume that a patient is brought to the x-ray department requiring, among other things, examination of the facial bones. We will further assume

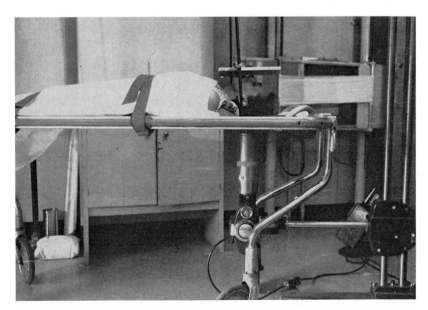

Fig. 11-10. A method for obtaining radiographs of facial bones through the stretcher top without physically positioning the patient.

that this patient, because of other injuries, cannot be removed from the x-ray stretcher. For evaluation of the facial bones, the Waters position and a lateral facial bone projection are desirable. A suggested procedure for obtaining a Waters position of the facial bones without moving the patient is as follows:

1. Place the portable x-ray machine in such a way that the tube is brought under the stretcher, pointing toward the ceiling of the room. Insert a cylinder cone into the aperture.

2. Position the x-ray tube and cone so that the usual Waters projection is covered.

3. Place rolled-up towels under the patient's shoulders and neck to permit the head to drop naturally into the "chin-nose" Waters position.

4. Place, on each side of the patient's skull, an ordinary laboratory pipette stand with clamps. Clamp the x-ray cassette onto the stand provided, and lower the cassette to the patient's chin.

Fig. 11-10 shows this position for the facial bones. Variations of the position can be used to obtain films of the zygomatic arch without moving the patient, using the cassette and the portable x-ray tube as the positioning variables. The cross-stretcher lateral films of the facial bones can be made on each side, using the same position variation shown in Fig. 11-3, illustrating lateral skull positions with corrected position of cassette and tube to cover the facial bones.

MISCELLANEOUS PRECAUTIONS TO BE OBSERVED BY THE X-RAY TECHNICIAN

The most common injury suffered by patients being admitted to emergency receiving departments is fracture of the extremities. There may be only a single fracture, or there may be multiple fractures. In textbooks on radiographic techniques, positioning for extremities is generally described in detail. In every instance the problem is approached with the idea of obtaining an ideal radiograph of a given part. In nearly ever instance, in order to obtain these ideal films, the technician is instructed to physically position the part under examination. However, it is usually wise to depart from these recommended methods when making x-ray examination on emergency patients suspected to have fractures. Until the nature and extent of the injuries are well defined, minimal handling of the patient by a technician is indicated.

The original film should be made to establish the character and extent of the injury so that a decision can be reached as to whether the textbook methods of positioning can be safely used. If possible, the injured part should not be moved at the start of the examination. Ingenuity on the part of the technician and flexibility of the x-ray equipment will usually permit several varied projections of an injured part without physically handling the part. Forcible positioning of a fractured extremity can result in further displacement of the fractured parts or even in compounding the fracture. After the original films have been viewed by the x-ray technician and the referring physician, a determination can be made as to whether the better projections described for examination of the part can be safely used.

It has been repeatedly emphasized that the physical positioning of the patient is usually contraindicated in a patient admitted for emergency treatment. Chest films may be required in a patient with heart failure. Such films should be made with the patient in a supine position, if his condition indicates no positioning or minimal positioning. If necessary, the film can be made with the patient in a semierect position, using the method described for an upright film of the abdomen.

The x-ray technician on an emergency service should be acquainted with special procedure equipment. An understanding of all the vascular radiographic procedures described in Chapter 9 is helpful. The technician may be called upon to do some of the special procedure examinations outlined in that chapter. It is not uncommon for patients admitted to emergency units to need immediate diagnostic procedures of the vascular type. These may be required because of traumatic injury to blood vessels or a rupture of a blood vessel. Many patients with this type of injury respond to the recently developed surgical techniques if the corrections are instituted immediately.

The challenge that exists to x-ray departments and their personnel as the result of the increase in emergency patients requiring x-ray examinations is difficult and complicated. Adequate flexible x-ray equipment and specially trained x-ray technicians seem to be the answer.

REFERENCES

1. Febboriello, M.: Personal communication, June 8, 1963.
2. MacEachern, M. T.: Hospital management and organization, ed. 3, Chicago, Physicians Record Co., pp. 343-345.

Chapter 12

Epilogue

Fiction writers often use the epilogue as a device to append the amplification or commentary of their works. Here the use of the device is to bring to the students' attention material that could not readily be allocated to the various chapters of this book without having the material appear somewhat out of context.

PATIENT CARE IN RADIATION THERAPY

It is probable that the patient admitted for radiation therapy treatment will present a different patient-care problem than the patient undergoing diagnostic x-ray examinations. He may be in poor condition physically and depressed mentally. A high percentage of radiation therapy patients have had recent surgery, and it is not unusual for this surgery to have been of a mutilating type. Aside from his attending physicians, nursing staff, and immediate family, the radiation therapists and technicians may be his first outside contacts since the operation. He will realize that the radiation therapist is a doctor concerned with his continued treatment. Intellectually, he may be able to accept the technical staff and receptionists in the therapy section in this way also. Practically, however, many patients will interpret the reaction of these new acquaintances as a sign of how he might expect to be received in the general public when finally discharged. The importance of the first impression he has as a patient in therapy cannot be overemphasized.

One of the main differences between patient care in diagnostic x-ray technology and radiation therapy technology is that the technician has a long contact with the patient over a period of time. One can readily see, therefore, how important it is to establish a good patient-technician relationship at the time of the first visit.

The postsurgical radiation therapy patient

Most patients in the postsurgical category have had their operation for the removal of some type of malignancy. Radiotherapy has been prescribed to ensure against metastasis (the transfer of the disease from a primary focus to a distant focus), to combat any malignant cells that might have remained following surgery, or in some instance, to treat areas that could not be corrected surgically. Often the patient will think that the surgery should have terminated his treatment. When the need for him to have continued treatment in the radiation therapy section is announced, the patient may become depressed and apprehensive. If the surgery has been a mutilating type requiring a good deal of adjustment on the part of the patient, his mental outlook toward his final recovery can be very pessimistic.

The mastectomy or radical mastectomy is a type of deforming surgery. A mastectomy is the surgical removal of a tumor of the breast. A radical mastectomy is the removal of the breast and a portion of the chest muscles and axillary lymph nodes. The patient who has had a mastectomy may feel that she has lost part of her identification as a woman. She further may feel that she has lost much of her physical attractiveness. She may think that people will find her unpleasant to look at.

She may not have been aware that a course in radiation therapy may be required following her surgery. Support and encouragement from all medical and technical personnel is vital in helping this patient gain a desire for recovery. A matter-of-fact attitude about her surgery by the technician and a pleasant manner can do much toward helping her. She will be uncomfortable when she comes to the department, not only at the surgical site but also throughout the shoulder and arm on the affected side. The technician should be aware that this patient must be encouraged to maintain good posture and that she probably has had instruction concerning exercise of the arm affected by the surgery.

As the technician will see this patient often and over a long period of time, it becomes important for the technician to encourage the patient in the use of the arm and, in fact, to remark in an encouraging fashion about the progress she is making that might be evidenced on each progressive visit.

Another type of deforming surgery that the technician in radiotherapy will see frequently is the patient with a colostomy. A colostomy is a surgical creation of an opening of the bowel so that it exits from the abdomen instead of the rectum. It is usually done because there is an obstruction and fecal material cannot go through the colon and into the rectum. Again, the patient who has had a colostomy may be very depressed and upset. He may have a difficult time accommodating to the new habits required of him and may feel very rejected and self-conscious. He might feel that any people, professional or otherwise, whom he meets will be offended because of the drainage problem that might exist. He realizes that his dietary habits have been changed and that he is faced for life with accommodating these changes.

Many malignancies of the head and neck will require radiation therapy following surgery. It is difficult for a patient to accept the changed appearance that occurs. The scars are obvious to everyone, and there is no way to camouflage them completely. He further may have great difficulty in eating and talking and will become very frustrated when he is not understood.

Radical surgery for tumors of the eye and sinuses are very deforming in appearance and, again, will contribute to patient dispair.

It is very important that the technician does not appear shocked or horrified when she encounters these patients. Her expression can easily convey this attitude. She must anticipate what the patient will look like and accept him as an ordinary person suffering from disease. An understanding of the surgical procedures some of these patients must undergo helps the technician in assisting the patients and understanding their individual needs.

Talking with the patient and, particularly, listening to the patient is very important. Conversation is therapeutic to the troubled person. It helps the patient reduce some of his anxieties about his disease and any fear of treatments he may have. The technician should make no attempt to dominate a conversation with the patient, but on the other hand, it is important to encourage these people to talk as this will open the door for reassurance to them. Most of all, the patient must be treated as an individual person and not as just another case requiring the use of hospital and your technical skills.

The nonsurgical radiation therapy patient

A wide variety of conditions are treated in the radiation therapy section in which the patient has not had preceding surgery. These patients fall into two general categories. In one instance, the patient is in radiation therapy for palliative treatment of some type, and in the other instance, for a variety of reasons, radiation therapy in some form is the treatment of choice.

The patient who comes to radiation therapy for palliative treatment often is a person with disease so advanced that a surgical approach is impossible. Psychologically, this patient is probably the most difficult to handle. Many times he is not aware of the fact that his disease may be terminal eventually. It is not unusual for him to be optimistic about the results of the treatment. The very fact that the patient has not had surgery may contribute to this optimistic feeling. Again, the technician must be careful not to contribute, by her attitude, anything that would further the optimism or, conversely, create an aura of apprehension.

It must be remembered that palliative treatment does relieve symptoms and can contribute to extended life. Often patients who come to the department for a course of treatment may be discharged only to be admitted some months later for a further course of treatment. If they have been the target of overoptimism at the time of the original series of treatments, the need for a second course of treatment might contribute to a deeper depression when this need occurs.

In the second general category, the patients whose disease dictates radiation therapy as the treatment of choice, a different technician attitude might be called for. Many types of malignant and nonmalignant skin diseases are included in this group. Patients will be concerned about their appearance; their disease may be causing considerable discomfort; their general health, however, may be good.

As is true in the patient with disfiguring surgery, it is important that the technician show no distaste or rejection in meeting and talking with the patient.

A condition which often faces the radiation therapy technician is the care of a patient who has as a primary source of disease malignant tumors involving the bone or metastatic disease to the bones. The physical handling of these patients is critical. Pathologic fractures can easily occur at the site of the disease in the bone with little or no external violence. Moving the patient from a stretcher to the therapy couch carelessly could cause this type of fracture. A pathologic fracture will cause the patient as much pain as an ordinary fracture and will be more difficult to treat.

As a general rule, the technician in radiation therapy must handle *all* patients carefully to avoid causing them discomfort, but in the care of the patient with bone disease, the added factor of causing the patient severe injury must be considered. The approach used by diagnostic x-ray technicians in handling the emergency patient with a spine injury is a similar problem.

THE PROBLEMS COMMON TO PATIENT CARE IN RADIATION THERAPY

The radiation therapy technician is often faced with inquiries from patients. They ask many questions about the results that they can expect from radiation therapy. They will inquire about treatment other than the treatments that they are receiving. All of this, of course, is a desperate subconscious probing for information as it relates to their own problems.

The technician must exercise extreme care during the course of these discussions. The patient's physicians have usually arrived at a decision as to what the patient should know and understand about his disease and about the treatment involved. It is not the technician's place to give out information that might be available to her about an individual patient's problem.

It is evident that the patients in radiation therapy have as primary problems fear, depression, apprehension, and discouragement. Many of the patients will be suffering discomfort or, in some cases, severe pain. Their introduction to the massive equipment (see Fig. 12-1) used in many of the treatments may cause them concern.

The fact that they are all alone in the room during treatment will tend to emphasize their concern. The problems in patient care of the radiation therapy patient are well known to most technicians but not necessarily easily solved.

It is not our purpose in this text to delve into the technical skills and knowledge a radiation therapy technician must have. It is our purpose to identify the care problems and suggest methods of combating them. The technician can be taught to physically handle a patient skillfully, provide comfort, maintain cleanliness, and even to show a superficial concern for others. The technician can acquire judgment to a degree and, with experience, learn to conceal undesirable emotions from others.

All of these skills will be exercised daily in the care of patients in a radiation therapy section. The ability to have genuine concern for others is probably a

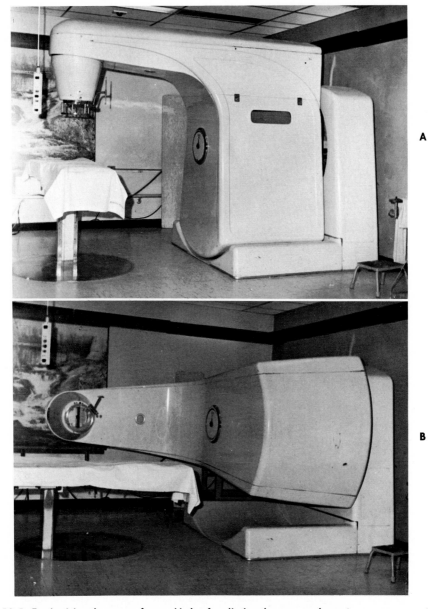

Fig. 12-1. Emphasizing the mass of some kinds of radiation therapy equipment.

product of a person's environment and heritage and is not an easily acquired trait. This ability, a therapy technician *must* have.

The key to proper care of the patient undergoing treatment lies in the technician's ability to gain the friendship, confidence, and respect of the person under treatment and to exercise careful judgment in communicating with him.

LYMPHANGIOGRAPHY

Lymphangiography is a technique for visualizing the lymph channels and nodes. It is usually done to detect metastatic malignant disease. The usual sterile technique procedures involving injection of contrast media must be followed.

A rather elaborate procedure must be followed in the lymphangiographic examination. As the lymph vessels are extremely small, it is not possible to readily identify them. The opening step in the examination involves injecting a blue dye beneath the skin. The dye is of a type that the lymph vessels will pick up readily and the radiologist then can observe their location and size. After the vessels are seen, a surgical incision is made over the vessel and an extremely small needle is placed in the lymph vessel. Following the introduction of the needle, a special type of pressure injector is attached, and under very slow and constant pressure, injection of the contrast material is begun. It usually takes about 1 hour to complete this injection.

At the end of the injection a set of films are made, and if the examination has been successful, the lymph channels will be visualized (see Fig. 12-2, *A*). The

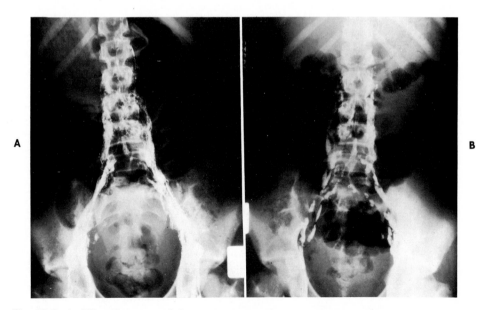

Fig. 12-2. A, Filling that occurs following injection in lymphangiography. **B,** 24-hour film demonstrating the continued presence but changed appearance of the contrast.

patient is then returned to his room, and about 24 hours later is brought back to the department for another set of films, and at this time the contrast medium will have concentrated in the lymph nodes (see Fig. 12-2, *B*).

Lymphangiography is really a small, delicate operation, and sterile precautions must be used. It is a long and tedious procedure for the patient as well as the radiologist. Every effort must be made to arrange the patient in a comfortable position. The injection is not necessarily made on the x-ray tables, because the patient can be readily transported to the x-ray table following the injection.

The intradermal injection of the blue dye which occurs at the beginning of the examination will cause the patient to have a bluish-green tinge to his skin for as long as 2 days. The patient should be aware of this possibility and should be reassured that it will go away and is not evidence of any disease or examination failure.

It is also wise for the technician to inform the nursing staff at the nursing station. The nurses in charge might not be aware of the possibility of a change in the patient's color which occurs during this procedure.

Index